Pocket Guide for

ECGs
MADE
EASY

Barbara Aehlert, MSEd, BSPA, RN

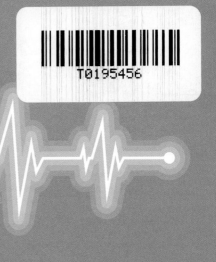

T0195456

ELSEVIER

Seventh Edition

ELSEVIER
3251 Riverport Lane
St. Louis, Missouri 63043

POCKET GUIDE FOR ECGs MADE EASY,
SEVENTH EDITION

ISBN: 978-0-323-83287-8

Notices

Knowledge and best practice in this field are constantly changing. As new research and experience broaden our understanding, changes in research methods, professional practices, or medical treatment may become necessary. Practitioners and researchers must always rely on their own experience and knowledge in evaluating and using any information, methods, compounds, or experiments described herein. In using such information or methods they should be mindful of their own safety and the safety of others, including parties for whom they have a professional responsibility. With respect to any drug or pharmaceutical products identified, readers are advised to check the most current information provided (i) on procedures featured or (ii) by the manufacturer of each product to be administered, to verify the recommended dose or formula, the method and duration of administration, and contraindications. It is the responsibility of practitioners, relying on their own experience and knowledge of their patients, to make diagnoses, to determine dosages and the best treatment for each individual patient, and to take all appropriate safety precautions.

To the fullest extent of the law, neither the Publisher nor the authors, contributors, or editors, assume any liability for any injury and/or damage to persons or property as a matter of products liability, negligence or otherwise, or from any use or operation of any methods, products, instructions, or ideas contained in the material herein.

Senior Content Strategist: Sandra Clark/Kelly Skelton
Content Development Manager: Laurie Gower
Senior Content Development Specialist: Elizabeth McCormac
Project Manager: Anne Collett
Design Direction: Brian Salisbury

Printed in Canada

Last digit is the print number: 9 8 7 6 5 4 3 2 1

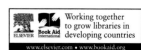

Working together
to grow libraries in
developing countries

www.elsevier.com • www.bookaid.org

Preface

This pocket guide is a handy, easy-to-use manual for interpretation of basic dysrhythmias. It's intended to accompany the seventh edition of the *ECGs Made Easy* textbook. In this reference, we've included a brief description of most of the rhythms discussed in the textbook. Each description is presented with a summary of rhythm characteristics and a sample rhythm strip.

All rhythm strips were recorded in lead II unless otherwise noted. Signs and symptoms associated with each rhythm, as well as treatment options, are outlined in the *ECGs Made Easy* textbook. We've made every attempt to provide information consistent with the current literature, including the latest resuscitation guidelines.

I genuinely hope this pocket guide is helpful to you, and I wish you success in your studies and clinical practice.

Best regards
Barbara Aehlert

Acknowledgments

I would like to thank the following healthcare professionals who provided many of the rhythm strips used in this book: Andrew Baird, CEP; James Bratcher; Joanna Burgan, CEP; Holly Button, CEP; Gretchen Chalmers, CEP; Thomas Cole, CEP; Brent Haines, CEP; Paul Honeywell, CEP; Timothy Klatt, RN; Bill Loughran, RN; Andrea Lowrey, RN; Joe Martinez, CEP; Stephanos Orphanidis, CEP; Jason Payne, CEP; Steve Ruehs, CEP; Patty Seneski, RN; David Stockton, CEP; Jason Stodghill, CEP; Dionne Socie, CEP; Kristina Tellez, CEP; and Fran Wojculewicz, RN.

About the Author

Barbara Aehlert, MSEd, BSPA, RN, has been a registered nurse for over 40 years, with clinical experience in medical/surgical nursing, critical care nursing, prehospital education, and nursing education.

Contents

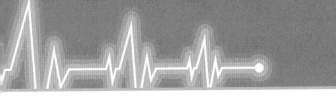
LOCATION, SIZE, AND SHAPE OF THE HEART

The heart is a hollow muscular organ that lies in the space between the lungs (i.e., the mediastinum) in the middle of the chest (Fig. 1.1). It sits behind the sternum and just above the diaphragm. About two-thirds of the heart lies to the left of the sternum's midline between the second and sixth ribs. The remaining third lies to the right of the sternum.

The adult heart is about the size of its owner's fist. The heart's weight is about 0.45% of a man's body weight and about 0.40% of a woman's. A person's heart size and weight are influenced by age, body weight and build, physical exercise frequency, and heart disease.

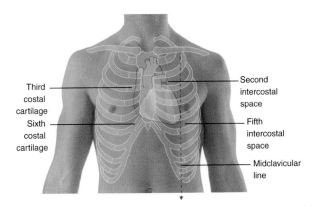

Fig. 1.1 Anterior view of the chest wall of a man showing skeletal structures and the surface projection of the heart. (From Drake R, Vogl AW, Mitchell AWM. *Gray's anatomy for students,* ed 3, New York, 2015, Churchill Livingstone.)

SURFACES OF THE HEART

The front (anterior) surface of the heart lies behind the sternum and costal cartilages. Most of the anterior surface is formed by the right atrium and the right ventricle, with the left ventricle contributing a small portion (Fig. 1.2). Because the heart is tilted slightly toward the left in the chest, the right ventricle is the heart area that lies most directly behind the sternum. The anterior surfaces of the right and left ventricles are separated by the left anterior descending artery (Gosling et al., 2017).

The heart's inferior surface, also called the diaphragmatic surface, is formed by the left and right ventricles and a small portion of the right atrium. The left ventricle makes up most of the inferior surface (Gosling et al., 2017).

The heart's base, or upper portion, is formed by the left atrium, a small portion of the right atrium, and portions of the superior and inferior venae cavae and the pulmonary veins (Fig. 1.3). The heart's

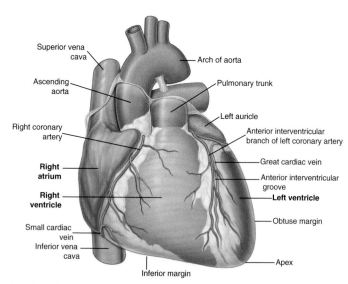

Fig. 1.2 The anterior surface of the heart. (From Drake R, Vogl AW, Mitchell AWM. *Gray's anatomy for students*, ed 3, New York, 2015, Churchill Livingstone.)

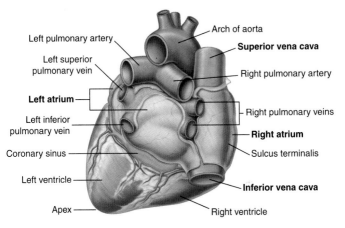

Fig. 1.3 The base of the heart. (From Drake R, Vogl AW, Mitchell AWM. *Gray's anatomy for students*, ed 3, New York, 2015, Churchill Livingstone.)

apex, or lower portion, is formed by the left ventricle's tip and is positioned at about the level of the left fifth intercostal space at the midclavicular line.

COVERINGS OF THE HEART

The *pericardium* is a double-walled sac that encloses the heart and helps protect it from trauma and infection. The pericardial sac's tough outer layer is called the fibrous parietal pericardium (Fig. 1.4). It anchors the heart to some of the structures around it, such as the sternum and diaphragm, through ligaments. This helps prevent excessive movement of the heart in the chest with changes in body position.

The pericardium's inner layer, the serous pericardium, consists of two layers: parietal and visceral. The parietal layer lines the inside of the fibrous pericardium. The visceral layer (i.e., the epicardium) attaches to the large vessels that enter and exit the heart and forms the heart's outer surface. Between the visceral and parietal layers is a space (the pericardial space) that generally contains about 20 mL of serous (pale yellow and transparent) fluid. This fluid acts as a lubricant, preventing friction as the heart beats.

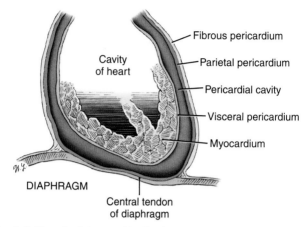

Fig. 1.4 The pericardial sac consists of two layers separated by a fluid-filled space. The visceral pericardium is attached directly to the heart's surface. The parietal pericardium forms the outer layer of the sac. (From Nagelhout JJ, Elisha S. *Nurse anesthesia*, ed 6, St. Louis, 2018, Elsevier.)

STRUCTURE OF THE HEART

Layers of the Heart Wall

The walls of the heart are made up of three tissue layers: the endocardium, myocardium, and epicardium. The heart's innermost layer, the *endocardium*, lines the heart's inner chambers, valves, chordae tendineae (tendinous cords), and papillary muscles. The endocardium is continuous with the innermost layer of the arteries, veins, and capillaries of the body, thereby creating a continuous, closed circulatory system. The *myocardium* (middle layer) is a thick, muscular layer that consists of cardiac muscle fibers (cells) responsible for the heart's pumping action. The heart's outermost layer is called the *epicardium* and contains blood capillaries, lymph capillaries, nerve fibers, and fat. The main coronary arteries lie on the epicardial surface of the heart. They feed this area first before entering the myocardium and supplying the heart's inner layers with oxygenated blood.

Cardiac Muscle

Cardiac muscle fibers make up the walls of the heart and surround the heart's chambers. Each muscle fiber is made up of many muscle cells.

Within each cell are mitochondria, the energy-producing parts of the cell, and bundles of myofibrils, which are long, tube-like structures packed closely together. Myofibrils are made up of many sarcomeres responsible for the contraction of muscle fibers and thousands of myofilaments. Each myofilament is made up of protein molecules. Myosin and actin are protein molecules that help to produce a contraction. Tropomyosin and troponin are protein molecules that inhibit myosin-actin interactions. When electrically stimulated, the contractile filaments slide together, changing the muscle fiber length and enabling contraction.

Intercalated disks join cardiac muscle cells together end to end. Gap junctions, which are like tunnels that join cell membranes, are present in the intercalated disks and allow electrical impulses to move rapidly from one fiber to another. The arrangement of the cardiac muscle fibers and intercalated disks allows cardiac muscle to function as a *syncytium*, which means that all fibers will become stimulated when one cardiac muscle fiber is stimulated (Koeppen & Stanton, 2018).

Heart Chambers

The heart has four chambers: two atria and two ventricles. The thickness of a heart chamber is related to the amount of pressure or resistance that the chamber's muscle must overcome to eject blood.

The heart's two upper chambers are the right and left atria (singular, *atrium*) (Fig. 1.5). Because the atria's purpose is to *receive* blood, think of them as holding tanks or reservoirs for blood for their respective ventricles. The right atrium receives blood low in oxygen from the superior vena cava (which carries blood from the head and upper extremities), the inferior vena cava (which carries blood from the lower body), and the coronary sinus (which is the largest vein that drains the heart). The left atrium receives freshly oxygenated blood from the lungs via the right and left pulmonary veins. The atria have thin walls because they encounter little resistance when pumping blood to the ventricles. Blood is pumped from the atria through an atrioventricular (AV) valve and into the ventricles.

The heart's two lower chambers are the right and left ventricles. Their purpose is to *pump* blood. The right ventricle pumps blood through the blood vessels of the lungs and then into the left atrium. The left ventricle pumps blood out to the body. Because the ventricles must pump blood either to the lungs (the right ventricle) or to the rest of the body (the left ventricle), the ventricles have a much thicker myocardial layer than the atria.

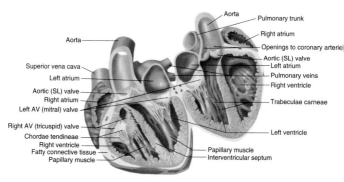

Fig. 1.5 Interior of the heart. This illustration shows the heart as it would appear if it were cut along a frontal plane and opened like a book. The heart's front portion lies to the reader's right; the back portion of the heart lies to the left. The four chambers of the heart—two atria and two ventricles—are easily seen. *AV*, atrioventricular; *SL*, semilunar. (From Patton KT, Thibodeau GA. *Anatomy & physiology*, ed 10, St. Louis, 2019, Elsevier.)

Heart Valves

There are four one-way valves in the heart: two AV valves and two semilunar (SL) valves (see Fig. 1.5). The valves open and close in a specific sequence and help produce the pressure gradient needed between the chambers to ensure a smooth flow of blood through the heart and prevent the backflow of blood.

AV valves separate the atria from the ventricles. The tricuspid valve is the AV valve that lies between the right atrium and right ventricle. It consists of three separate cusps or flaps. It is larger in diameter and thinner than the mitral valve. The mitral (or bicuspid) valve has only two cusps. It lies between the left atrium and left ventricle.

The pulmonic and aortic valves are SL valves. The SL valves prevent backflow of blood from the aorta and pulmonary arteries into the ventricles. The SL valves have three cusps, shaped like half-moons. The SL valves' openings are smaller than the AV valves' openings, and the flaps of the SL valves are smaller and thicker than the AV valves.

Heart sounds occur because of vibrations in the heart's tissues caused by the closing of the heart's valves. Vibrations are created as blood flow is suddenly increased or slowed with the contraction and relaxation of the heart chambers and with the opening and closing of the valves. The first heart sound, known as S_1, is the result of closure of the tricuspid and mitral (AV) valves and reflects the start of ventricular contraction. The second heart sound (i.e., S_2) is caused by closure of the pulmonic and aortic (SL) valves and reflects the start of ventricular relaxation.

THE HEART'S BLOOD SUPPLY

The main coronary arteries lie on the outer (i.e., epicardial) surface of the heart. Coronary arteries that run on the surface of the heart are called epicardial coronary arteries. They branch into progressively smaller vessels, eventually becoming arterioles and then capillaries.

The three major epicardial coronary arteries include the left anterior descending (LAD) artery, circumflex (Cx) artery, and right coronary artery (RCA) (Fig. 1.6, Table 1.1). A person is said to have coronary artery disease (CAD) if there is more than 50% diameter narrowing (i.e., stenosis) in one or more of these vessels.

The coronary (cardiac) veins travel alongside the arteries. The coronary sinus is the largest vein that drains the heart. It receives blood from the great, middle, and small cardiac veins; a vein of the left atrium; and the left ventricle's posterior vein. The coronary sinus drains into the right atrium.

Acute Coronary Syndromes

Acute coronary syndrome (ACS) is a term that refers to distinct conditions caused by a similar sequence of pathologic events involving abruptly reduced coronary artery blood flow. This sequence of events results in conditions that range from myocardial ischemia or injury to death (i.e., necrosis) of the heart muscle.

The usual cause of an ACS is the rupture of an atherosclerotic plaque. Arteriosclerosis is a chronic disease of the arterial system characterized by abnormal thickening and hardening of the vessel walls. Atherosclerosis is a form of arteriosclerosis. The thickening and hardening of the vessel walls are caused by a buildup of fat-like deposits (e.g., plaque) in the inner lining of large and middle-sized muscular arteries. As the fatty deposits build up, the artery's opening slowly narrows, and blood flow to the muscle decreases. The extent of arterial narrowing and the amount of blood flow reduction are critical determinants of coronary artery disease.

Angina pectoris is chest discomfort or other related symptoms that occur suddenly when the heart's increased oxygen demand temporarily exceeds the blood supply. Angina is a symptom of myocardial ischemia,

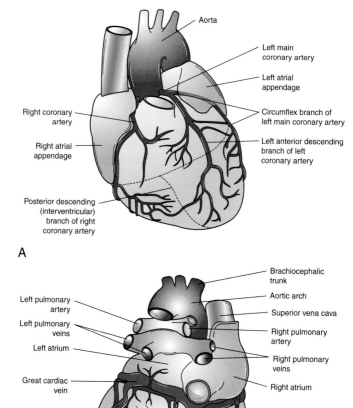

Fig. 1.6 Coronary arteries supplying the heart. The right coronary artery supplies the right atrium, ventricle, and posterior aspect of the left ventricle in most individuals. The left coronary artery divides into the left anterior descending and circumflex arteries, which perfuse the left ventricle. **A**, Anterior view. **B**, Posterior view. (From Banasik JL, Copstead LC, Banasik JL. *Pathophysiology*, ed 6, St. Louis, 2019, Elsevier.)

TABLE 1.1	Coronary Arteries	
Coronary Artery	Portion of Myocardium Supplied	Portion of Conduction System Supplied
Right	• Right atrium • Right ventricle • Inferior surface of left ventricle (about 85%)[a] • Posterior surface of left ventricle (85%)[a]	• Sinoatrial (SA) node (about 60%)[a] • Atrioventricular (AV) bundle (85% to 90%)[a]
Left anterior descending	• Anterior surface of left ventricle • Part of lateral surface of left ventricle • Anterior two-thirds of interventricular septum	• Most of right bundle branch • Part of left bundle branch
Circumflex	• Left atrium • Part of lateral surface of left ventricle • Inferior surface of left ventricle (about 15%)[a] • Posterior surface of left ventricle (15%)[a]	• SA node (about 40%)[a] • AV bundle (10% to 15%)[a]

[a]Percentage of the population.

and it most often occurs in patients with CAD that involves at least one coronary artery. However, it can be present in patients with normal coronary arteries. Angina also occurs in people with uncontrolled high blood pressure or valvular heart disease.

Partial or intermittent blockage of a coronary artery may result in no clinical symptoms (i.e., silent ischemia), angina, a heart attack, which is also called a *myocardial infarction (MI)*, or sudden death. The area supplied by a blocked coronary artery goes through a sequence of events that have been identified as zones of ischemia, injury, and infarction. Each zone is associated with characteristic ECG changes. When myocardial ischemia or infarction is suspected, an understanding of coronary artery anatomy and the heart areas that each vessel supplies helps you predict which coronary artery is blocked and anticipate problems associated with blockage of that vessel.

If the blocked coronary vessel is quickly opened to restore blood flow and oxygen to the injured area, no tissue death occurs. Methods of restoring blood flow may include giving clot-busting drugs (i.e., fibrinolytics) or performing endovascular therapies.

THE HEART'S NERVE SUPPLY

Both divisions of the autonomic nervous system innervate fibers to the heart. The sympathetic division prepares the body to function under stress (i.e., the "fight-or-flight" response). The parasympathetic division conserves and restores body resources (i.e., the "rest and digest" response).

Sympathetic (accelerator) nerves innervate specific areas of the heart's electrical system, atrial muscle, and the ventricular myocardium. When sympathetic nerves are stimulated, the neurotransmitters norepinephrine and epinephrine are released resulting in an increased heart rate, force of contraction, conduction velocity, blood pressure, and cardiac output.

Parasympathetic (inhibitory) nerve fibers innervate the sinoatrial (SA) node, atrial muscle, and the heart's AV bundle by the vagus nerves. Acetylcholine is a chemical messenger (neurotransmitter) released when parasympathetic nerves are stimulated. Parasympathetic stimulation slows the rate of discharge of the SA node, slows conduction through the AV node, decreases the strength of atrial contraction, and can cause a small decrease in the force of ventricular contraction.

THE HEART AS A PUMP

The right and left sides of the heart are separated by an internal wall of connective tissue called a *septum*. The *interatrial septum* separates the right and left atria. The *interventricular septum* separates the right and left ventricles. The septa separate the heart into two functional pumps. The right atrium and right ventricle make up one pump. The left atrium and left ventricle make up the other (Fig. 1.7). The heart's right side, called the pulmonary circulation, is a low-pressure system whose job is to pump unoxygenated blood from the body to and through the lungs to the left side of the heart. The heart's left side, called the systemic circulation, receives oxygenated blood from the lungs and pumps it out to the rest of the body. Blood is carried from the heart to the body's organs through arteries, arterioles, and capillaries. Blood is returned to the right side of the heart through venules and veins.

Cardiac Cycle

The cardiac cycle refers to a repetitive pumping process that includes all of the events associated with blood flow through the heart. The cycle has two phases for each heart chamber: systole and diastole. *Systole* is

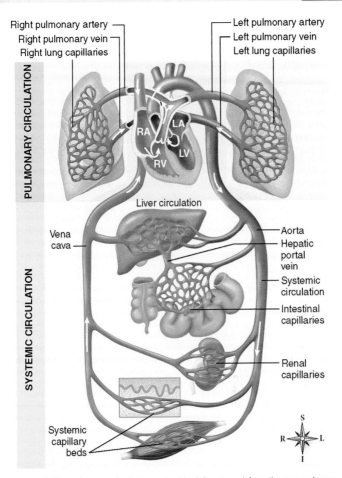

Fig. 1.7 The pulmonary circulation routes blood flow to and from the gas-exchange tissues of the lungs. The systemic circulation routes blood flow to and from the oxygen-consuming tissues of the body. *LA*, left atrium; *LV*, left ventricle; *RA*, right atrium; *RV*, right ventricle. (From Patton KT, Thibodeau GA. *Anthony's textbook of anatomy and physiology*, ed 21, St. Louis, 2019, Elsevier.)

the period during which the chamber contracts and blood is ejected. *Diastole* is the period of relaxation during which the chambers fill. The myocardium receives its fresh supply of oxygenated blood from the coronary arteries during ventricular diastole.

During the cardiac cycle, the pressure within each chamber of the heart rises in systole and falls in diastole. The heart's valves ensure that blood flows in the proper direction. Blood flows from one heart chamber to another from higher to lower pressure. These pressure relationships depend on the careful timing of contractions. The heart's conduction system provides the necessary timing of events between atrial and ventricular systole.

Blood from the tissues of the head, neck, and upper extremities is emptied into the superior vena cava. Blood from the lower body is returned to the inferior vena cava. During atrial diastole, blood from the superior and inferior vena cavae and the coronary sinus enters the right atrium. The right atrium fills and distends. This pushes the tricuspid valve open and the right ventricle fills. The left atrium receives oxygenated blood from the four pulmonary veins (two from the right lung and two from the left lung). The mitral valve flaps open as the left atrium fills, allowing blood to flow into the left ventricle.

As the ventricles contract, blood is propelled through the systemic and pulmonary circulation and toward the atria. When the right ventricle contracts, the tricuspid valve closes. The right ventricle expels the blood through the pulmonic valve into the pulmonary trunk. The pulmonary trunk divides into a right and left pulmonary artery, each of which carries blood to one lung (i.e., the pulmonary circuit). Blood flows through the pulmonary arteries to the lungs. Blood low in oxygen passes through the pulmonary capillaries. There it comes in direct contact with the alveolar-capillary membrane, where oxygen and carbon dioxide are exchanged. Blood then flows into the pulmonary veins and then to the left atrium.

When the left ventricle contracts, the mitral valve closes to prevent backflow of blood. Blood leaves the left ventricle through the aortic valve to the aorta, which is the main vessel of the systemic arterial circulation. Blood is distributed throughout the body (i.e., the systemic circuit) through the aorta and its branches. Blood continues to move in one direction because pressure pushes it from the high-pressure (i.e., arterial) side, and valves in the veins prevent backflow on the lower pressure (i.e., venous) side as blood returns to the heart.

Blood Pressure

The pulse and blood pressure reflect the mechanical activity of the heart. *Blood pressure* (BP) is the force exerted by the circulating blood volume on the walls of the arteries. The volume of blood in the arteries is directly related to arterial blood pressure. Blood pressure is equal to cardiac output × peripheral resistance. *Peripheral resistance* is the resistance to the flow of blood determined by blood vessel diameter and the tone of the vascular musculature. Blood pressure is affected by conditions or medications that alter peripheral resistance or cardiac output.

Cardiac output (CO) is the amount of blood pumped into the aorta each minute by the left ventricle (Pappano & Wier, 2019). Four factors determine CO: heart rate (HR), myocardial contractility, preload, and afterload. CO is defined as the *stroke volume (SV)*, which is the amount of blood ejected from the left ventricle with each heartbeat, multiplied by the HR. Increases in HR shorten all phases of the cardiac cycle, including the time the ventricles spend relaxing. If the length of time for ventricular relaxation is shortened, there is less time for them to fill adequately with blood.

Each ventricle holds about 150 mL of blood when it is full. They usually eject about half this volume (70 to 80 mL) with each contraction. In a healthy average adult, the CO at rest is about 5 L/min. The percentage of blood pumped out of a ventricle with each contraction is called the *ejection fraction*. Ejection fraction is used as a measure of ventricular function.

REFERENCES

Gosling, J. A., Harris, P. F., Humpherson, J. R., Whitmore, I., & Willan, P. L. (2017). Thorax. In J. A. Gosling, P. F. Harris, J. R. Humpherson, I. Whitmore, & P. L. Willan (Eds.), *Human anatomy, color atlas and textbook* (6 ed., pp. 25–70). London: Elsevier.

Koeppen, B. M., & Stanton, B. A. (2018). Elements of cardiac function. In B. M. Koeppen & B. A. Stanton (Eds.), *Berne & Levy physiology* (7 ed., pp. 304–344). Philadelphia, PA: Elsevier.

Pappano, A. J., & Wier, W. G. (2019). Control of cardiac output: *In Cardiovascular physiology* (11 ed., pp. 176–200). Philadelphia, PA: Elsevier.

CARDIAC CELLS

Types of Cardiac Cells

In general, cardiac cells have either a mechanical (i.e., contractile) or an electrical (i.e., pacemaker) function. *Myocardial cells* contain contractile filaments. When these cells are electrically stimulated, these filaments slide together and cause the myocardial cell to contract. These myocardial cells form the thin muscular layer of the atrial walls and the thicker muscular layer of the ventricular walls (i.e., the myocardium).

Pacemaker cells are specialized cells of the electrical conduction system that can form electrical impulses spontaneously and can alter the speed of electrical conduction (Wagner, 2012).

Properties of Cardiac Cells

The heart's pacemaker cells can generate an electrical impulse without being stimulated from another source. This property is called *automaticity*. Cardiac muscle is electrically irritable because of an ionic imbalance across the membranes of cells. *Excitability* (i.e., irritability) is a cardiac cell's ability to respond to a stimulus, such as a chemical, mechanical, or electrical source. *Conductivity* is a cardiac cell's ability to receive an electrical impulse and conduct it to an adjacent cardiac cell. All cardiac cells possess this characteristic. The intercalated disks present in the membranes of cardiac cells are responsible for the property of conductivity. They allow an impulse in any part of the myocardium to spread throughout the heart. The speed with which the impulse is conducted can be altered by sympathetic and parasympathetic stimulation and medications. *Contractility* (i.e., inotropy) is myocardial cells' ability to shorten, thereby causing cardiac muscle contraction in response to an electrical stimulus. The strength of the heart's contraction can be increased or decreased with certain medications.

CARDIAC ACTION POTENTIAL

Human body fluids contain electrolytes, which are elements or compounds that break into charged particles (i.e., ions) when melted or dissolved in water or another solvent. Differences in the composition of ions between the intracellular and extracellular fluid compartments are essential for normal body function, including the heart's activity.

In the body, ions spend much time moving back and forth across cell membranes. As a result, a slight difference in the concentrations of charged particles across the membranes of cells is normal; thus, potential energy (i.e., voltage) exists because of the imbalance of charged particles. This imbalance makes the cells excitable. The voltage (i.e., the difference in electrical charges) across the cell membrane is the membrane potential. The threshold potential is the voltage level at which the cell discharges and conducts an electrical impulse.

Electrolytes are quickly moved from one side of the cell membrane to the other using pumps. These pumps require energy in the form of adenosine triphosphate (ATP) when movement occurs against a concentration gradient. The energy expended by the cells to move electrolytes across the cell membrane creates a flow of current. This flow of current is expressed in volts or millivolts (mV). Voltage appears on an electrocardiogram (ECG) as waveforms. A cardiac cell's *action potential* reflects the rapid sequence of voltage changes across the cell membrane during the electrical cardiac cycle.

Depolarization and Repolarization

Depolarization is the movement of ions across a cell membrane, causing the inside of the cell to become more positive. Depolarization, an electrical event, must occur before the heart can contract and pump blood, which is a mechanical event. The stimulus that alters the electrical charges across the cell membrane may be electrical, mechanical, or chemical. An impulse normally begins in the pacemaker cells found in the sinoatrial (SA) node of the heart. A chain reaction (a wave of depolarization) occurs from cell to cell in the heart's electrical conduction system until all the cells have been stimulated and

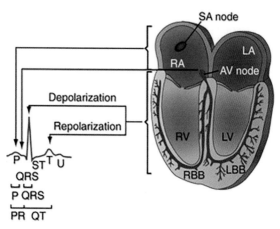

Fig. 2.1 Schematic representation of the electrocardiogram and its relationship to cardiac electrical activity. *AV*, atrioventricular; *LA*, left atrium; *LBB*, left bundle branch; *LV*, left ventricle; *RA*, right atrium; *RBB*, right bundle branch; *RV*, right ventricle; *SA*, sinoatrial. (From McCance KL, Huether SE. *Pathophysiology*, ed 8, St. Louis, 2019, Elsevier.)

depolarized. The chain reaction is made possible because of the gap junctions that exist between the cells. These junctions permit ions to flow from one cell into the next. Eventually, the impulse is spread from the pacemaker cells to the working myocardial cells, which contract when stimulated.

After the cell depolarizes, it quickly begins to recover and restore its electrical charges to normal. The movement of charged particles across a cell membrane in which the inside of the cell is restored to its negative charge is called *repolarization*. As the cell returns to its polarized (i.e., resting) state, contractile proteins in the working myocardial cells separate (i.e., relax). The cell can be stimulated again if another electrical impulse arrives at the cell membrane (Fig. 2.1).

Action Potentials

There are two main types of action potentials in the heart: fast potentials and slow potentials. The action potential configuration varies depending on the cardiac cell's location and function (Fig. 2.2). The fast response action potential occurs in atrial and ventricular working

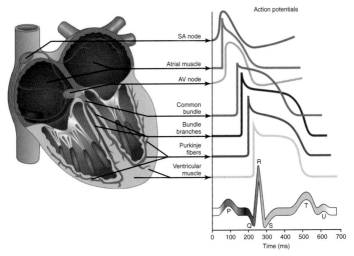

Fig. 2.2 Cardiac action potentials from the sinoatrial node to the ventricular myocardium. *AV*, atrioventricular; *SA*, sinoatrial. (From Dowd FJ, Johnson BS, Mariotti AJ. *Pharmacology and therapeutics for dentistry*, ed 7, St. Louis, 2017, Elsevier.)

myocardial cells and His–Purkinje fibers (Issa et al., 2019), which are specialized conducting fibers. The cardiac action potential is divided into several phases, which reflect the permeability of the cell membrane to different electrolytes. The second type of cardiac action potential, the slow response action potential, occurs in the heart's normal pacemaker (i.e., the SA node) and in the atrioventricular (AV) node, which is the specialized conducting tissue that carries an electrical impulse from the atria to the ventricles.

REFRACTORY PERIODS

Excitability is the ability of myocardial cells to respond to a stimulus. The excitability of a myocardial cell varies throughout the action potential, and these changes in excitability are reflected in refractory periods (Costanzo, 2018).

Refractoriness is a term used to describe the period of recovery that cells need after being discharged before they are once again able to respond to a stimulus. The *effective refractory period (ERP)*, also called the *absolute refractory period*, is the interval from the beginning of

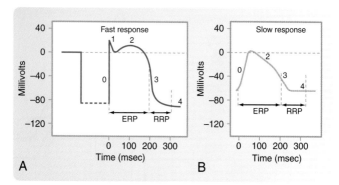

Fig. 2.3 Action potentials of fast-response (**A**) and slow-response (**B**) cardiac fibers. The phases of the action potentials are labeled. The effective refractory period (ERP) and the relative refractory period (RRP) are labeled. Note that when compared with fast-response fibers, the resting potential of slow fibers is less negative, the upstroke (phase 0) of the action potential is less steep, the amplitude of the action potential is smaller, phase 1 is absent, and the RRP extends well into phase 4 after the fibers have fully repolarized. (From Koeppen BM, Stanton BA. *Berne & Levy physiology*, ed 7, Philadelphia, 2018, Elsevier.)

the action potential until the myocardial fiber can conduct another action potential (Pappano & Wier, 2019). The *relative refractory period (RRP)* begins at the end of the ERP and ends when the cell membrane is almost entirely repolarized (Fig. 2.3). During the RRP, some cardiac cells have repolarized to their threshold potential and thus can be stimulated to respond (i.e., depolarize) to a stronger-than-normal stimulus.

CONDUCTION SYSTEM

The specialized electrical (i.e., pacemaker) cells in the heart are arranged in a system of pathways called the *conduction system* (Fig. 2.4, Table 2.1). In the normal heart, the cells of the conduction system are interconnected. The conduction system ensures that the chambers of the heart contract in a coordinated fashion.

CAUSES OF DYSRHYTHMIAS

Dysrhythmias result from disorders of impulse formation, disorders of impulse conduction, or both.

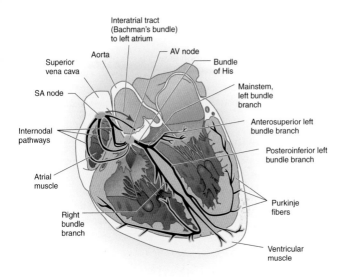

Fig. 2.4 Conduction pathways through the heart. A section through the long axis of the heart is shown. *AV*, atrioventricular; *SA*, sinoatrial. (From Boron WF, Boulpaep EL. *Medical physiology*, ed 3, Philadelphia, 2017, Elsevier.)

TABLE **2.1**	Summary of the Conduction System	
Structure	**Function**	**Intrinsic Pacemaker (beats/min)**
Sinoatrial (SA) node	Primary pacemaker; initiates impulse that is normally conducted throughout the left and right atria	60 to 100
Atrioventricular (AV) node	Receives impulse from the SA node and delays the relay of the impulse to the bundle of His	
Bundle of His (AV bundle)	Receives impulse from the AV node and relays it to the right and left bundle branches	40 to 60
Right and left bundle branches	Receives impulse from the bundle of His and relays it to the Purkinje fibers	
Purkinje fibers	Receives impulse from the bundle branches and relays it to the ventricular myocardium	20 to 40

Disorders of Impulse Formation

Altered Automaticity

Altered automaticity is a condition in which one of the following occurs: (1) cardiac cells that are generally not associated with a pacemaker function begin to depolarize spontaneously *or* (2) a pacemaker site other than the SA node increases its firing rate beyond that which is considered normal.

Triggered Activity

Triggered activity occurs when escape pacemaker and working cells fire more than once after stimulation by a single impulse. It results from abnormal electrical impulses that sometimes occur during repolarization (i.e., afterdepolarizations) when cells are normally quiet. Triggered activity can result in atrial or ventricular beats that occur alone, in pairs, in runs of three or more beats, or as a sustained ectopic rhythm.

Disorders of Impulse Conduction

Conduction Blocks

Blockage of impulse conduction may be partial or complete. A block may occur because of trauma, drug toxicity, electrolyte disturbances, myocardial ischemia, or infarction. A partial conduction block may cause the impulse to become slowed or intermittent. In slowed conduction, all impulses are conducted, but it takes longer than normal to do so. When an intermittent block occurs, some (but not all) impulses are conducted. When a complete block exists, no impulses are conducted through the affected area.

Reentry

Usually, an impulse spreads through the heart only once after it is initiated by pacemaker cells. When *reentry* occurs, also called *reactivation*, an electrical impulse is delayed, blocked, or both in one or more areas of the conduction system while being conducted normally through the rest of the system. This results in the delayed electrical impulse entering cardiac cells that the normally conducted impulse has just depolarized. Reentry requires the following three conditions: (1) an area of unidirectional conduction block, (2) an area of delayed conduction, and (3) an area of unexcitable tissue (Peterson, 2018).

THE ELECTROCARDIOGRAM

The electrocardiogram (ECG) is a graphic display of the heart's electrical activity. When electrodes are attached to the patient's limbs or chest and connected by cables to an ECG machine, the ECG machine functions as a voltmeter, detecting and recording the voltage changes (i.e., action potentials) generated by depolarization and repolarization of the heart's cells. The voltage changes are displayed as specific waveforms and complexes (Fig. 2.5).

The ECG can provide information about the following:

- The orientation of the heart in the chest
- Conduction disturbances
- Electrical effects of medications and electrolytes
- The mass of cardiac muscle
- The presence of ischemic damage

The ECG does *not* provide information about the mechanical (contractile) condition of the myocardium. Assess the patient's pulse and blood pressure to evaluate the effectiveness of the heart's mechanical activity.

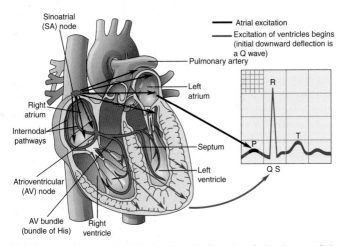

Fig. 2.5 Schematic drawing of the heart's conduction system. An impulse normally is generated in the sinoatrial node. It travels through the atria to the atrioventricular node, down the bundle of His and Purkinje fibers, and to the ventricular myocardium. Recording of the depolarizing and repolarizing currents in the heart with electrodes on the body's surface produces characteristic waveforms. (From Copstead-Kirkhorn LE, Banasik JL. *Pathophysiology*, ed 5, St. Louis, 2013, Saunders.)

Electrodes

Electrode refers to an adhesive pad containing a conductive substance in the center applied to the patient's skin. The electrode's conductive media conducts skin surface voltage changes through wires to a cardiac monitor (i.e., electrocardiograph). Electrodes are applied at specific locations on the patient's chest wall and extremities to view the heart's electrical activity from different angles and planes. One end of a monitoring cable, also called a lead wire, is attached to the electrode and the other to an ECG machine. The cable conducts current back to the cardiac monitor. ECG cables may be coded by color, symbol, or letter. However, colors are not standard and often vary.

Leads

A *lead* is a record (i.e., tracing) of electrical activity between two electrodes. Each lead records the *average* current flow at a specific time in a portion of the heart. Leads allow for viewing the heart's electrical activity in the frontal and horizontal (transverse) planes (Fig. 2.6). A 12-lead ECG views the heart in both the frontal and horizontal planes and views the left ventricle's surfaces from multiple angles. The 12-lead ECG is a useful diagnostic study you can obtain when there are changes in a patient's cardiac rhythm or condition. Six leads view the heart in the frontal plane. Leads I, II, and III are called *standard limb leads*. Leads aVR, aVL, and aVF are called *augmented limb leads*. Six chest (i.e., precordial or "V") leads view the heart in the horizontal plane, allowing views of the front and left side of the heart. A summary of the standard limb leads can be found in Table 2.2, a summary of the augmented leads appears in Table 2.3, and a summary of the chest leads appears in Table 2.4.

Right Chest Leads

Other chest leads that are not part of a standard 12-lead ECG reveal specific surfaces of the heart. Right chest leads are used to evaluate the right ventricle (Fig. 2.7). Right chest lead placement is identical to standard chest lead placement, except that it is done on the chest's right side. Obtain a standard 12-lead ECG first; then reposition the electrodes on the right side of the chest and attach the cables for the standard chest leads to the repositioned electrodes to obtain the additional leads. If time does not permit obtaining all of the right chest leads, the lead of choice is V_4R.

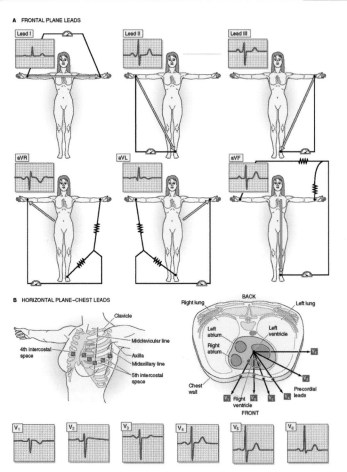

Fig. 2.6 The electrocardiogram (ECG) leads. (From Boron WF, Boulpaep EL. *Medical physiology*, ed 3, Philadelphia, 2017, Elsevier.)

TABLE 2.2	Standard Limb Leads		
Lead	Positive Electrode	Negative Electrode	Heart Surface Viewed
I	Left arm	Right arm	Lateral
II	Left leg	Right arm	Inferior
III	Left leg	Left arm	Inferior

TABLE **2.3**	Augmented Leads	
Lead	Positive Electrode	Heart Surface Viewed
aVR	Right arm	None
aVL	Left arm	Lateral
aVF	Left leg	Inferior

TABLE **2.4**	Chest Leads	
Lead	Positive Electrode Position	Heart Surface Viewed
V_1	Right side of sternum, fourth intercostal space	Interventricular septum
V_2	Left side of sternum, fourth intercostal space	Interventricular septum
V_3	Midway between V_2 and V_4	Anterior surface
V_4	Left midclavicular line, fifth intercostal space	Anterior surface
V_5	Left anterior axillary line; same level as V_4	Lateral surface
V_6	Left midaxillary line; fifth intercostal space	Lateral surface

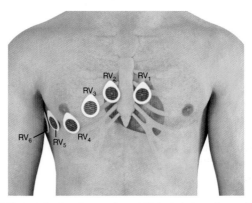

Fig. 2.7 Electrode locations for recording a right chest electrocardiogram (ECG). Right chest leads are used when a right ventricular infarction is suspected. (From Roberts JR, Custalow CB, Thomsen TW. *Roberts and Hedges' clinical procedures in emergency medicine and acute care*, ed 7, Philadelphia, 2019, Elsevier.)

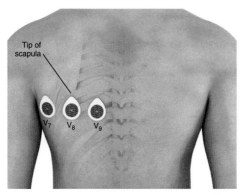

Fig. 2.8 Electrode locations for left posterior chest lead placement. (From Roberts JR, Custalow CB, Thomsen TW. *Roberts and Hedges' clinical procedures in emergency medicine and acute care*, ed 7, Philadelphia, 2019, Elsevier.)

Posterior Chest Leads

On a standard 12-lead ECG, no leads look directly at the posterior surface of the heart. Additional chest leads may be used for this purpose. These leads are placed farther left and toward the back. All the leads are placed on the same horizontal line as V_4 to V_6. Lead V_7 is placed at the posterior axillary line. Lead V_8 is placed at the angle of the scapula (i.e., the posterior scapular line), and lead V_9 is placed over the left border of the spine (Fig. 2.8).

Ambulatory Cardiac Monitoring

Ambulatory cardiac monitoring, also known as ambulatory electrocardiographic (AECG) monitoring, is a noninvasive diagnostic tool used to monitor the patient's cardiac rhythm as they perform daily activities. Examples of indications for AECG monitoring include the following:

- To determine the association between a patient's symptoms (e.g., dizziness, palpitations, near syncope, shortness of breath, chest pain, fatigue) and cardiac rhythm disturbances
- To detect myocardial ischemia and to evaluate the efficacy of anti-ischemic medications in patients with coronary artery disease
- To assess the patient's risk of dysrhythmias after myocardial infarction; for patients with heart failure, hypertrophic cardiomyopathy, diabetic neuropathy, systemic hypertension, or valvular heart

disease; for patients receiving hemodialysis; and for the preoperative evaluation of patients and after cardiac operations

- To assess the efficacy of medications on the cardiac conduction system, the patient's cardiac rhythm, or both
- To aid in correlating patient symptoms with dysrhythmias and evaluating symptomatic patients for pacemaker implantation
- To assess the function of implanted devices, such as a pacemaker or an implantable cardioverter-defibrillator
- To assess the efficacy of ablation procedures

Several types of devices are used for AECG monitoring. The choice of equipment used is based on the frequency of the patient's symptoms. A Holter monitor is a battery-powered continuous AECG recorder used when patient symptoms occur often enough to be detected during a short period (24 hours to 72 hours) of monitoring. Holter monitors continuously record at least 2 leads, and newer models can record and store up to 2 weeks of data. Electrodes and lead wires are connected to a portable, lightweight recorder attached to the patient and carried with a belt or shoulder strap. When the monitoring period is complete, the patient returns the monitor and events that have been stored on a digital flash memory device that is then scanned by a technician and interpreted by a physician. This information is then compared with the ECG events captured by the device to determine if a relationship exists among the patient's symptoms, activities, and ECG.

An event monitor is a portable recording device that intermittently records and stores ECG data for 14 to 30 days or longer. It is used when the patient's symptoms are unlikely to be captured during a 24- to 72-hour period.

An external loop recorder, also called a *looping memory monitor*, continuously records and stores ECG data over weeks to months. It is used when the patient's symptoms are likely to recur within a 2- to 6-week period. The recorder is connected to the patient using electrodes and lead wires. The device stores a single external modified limb lead ECG with a 4- to 60-minute memory buffer (Krahn et al., 2018). When a patient experiences symptoms, they activate the device, which stores the previous 3 to 14 minutes of recorded data before the event. Also, 1 to 4 minutes of data are recorded and stored after the triggered event. The captured data can subsequently be uploaded and analyzed, often providing critical information regarding the onset and termination of the dysrhythmia (Krahn et al., 2018).

External patch recorders permit ECG monitoring, typically for 7 to 14 days. The device has no leads or wires; an adhesive is used to attach it to the patient's chest wall. With one type of patch-based recording system, data are recorded continuously and then later analyzed. Another patch-based recording system uses Bluetooth technology to transmit data in real-time using a smartphone-like device carried by the patient. The data is then transmitted to a central monitoring center, where it is analyzed and interpreted by trained clinicians (Krahn et al., 2018).

Mobile cardiac outpatient telemetry is used when a patient's symptoms are infrequent. It is a real-time monitoring system that automatically gathers data from a patch applied to the patient's skin and an attached sensor using Bluetooth technology. When a dysrhythmia is detected, the device transmits the ECG data to a receiving center staffed with trained technicians.

An implantable loop recorder, also called an insertable cardiac monitor, is a small ECG recording device that resembles a flash drive. It is used when a patient's symptoms (e.g., fainting, seizures, palpitations) are recurrent but infrequent. An insertable monitor is usually implanted under the skin on the left chest under local anesthesia. The device records a single ECG lead and has a battery life of 2 to 3 years (Shen et al., 2017). The patient or a family member can manually activate the device with a small, handheld activator placed on the chest wall over the monitor when the patient experiences symptoms.

Several portable handheld ECG monitors are available for home use. Most handheld ECG monitors record in a single limb lead, and some display the ECG rhythm while recording.

Electrocardiography Paper

When you place electrodes on the patient's body and connect them to an electrocardiograph, the machine records the voltage (i.e., the potential difference) between the electrodes. The needle, or pen, of the ECG moves a specific distance depending on the voltage measured. This recording is made on ECG paper.

ECG paper is graph paper made up of small and large boxes measured in millimeters. The smallest boxes are 1 mm wide and 1 mm high (Fig. 2.9). The horizontal axis of the paper corresponds with time. Time is used to measure the duration of specific cardiac events, which is stated in seconds. Measuring how quickly or slowly an electrical impulse spreads through the heart provides essential information about the condition of the heart's conduction system and the muscle itself.

ECG paper normally records at a constant speed of 25 mm/second. Thus, each horizontal unit (i.e., each 1-mm box) represents 0.04 second

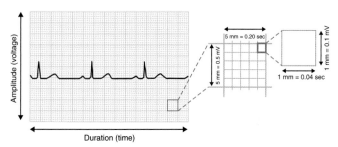

Fig. 2.9 Electrocardiographic strip showing the markings for measuring amplitude and duration of waveforms, using a standard recording speed of 25 mm/second. (From Copstead-Kirkhorn LE, Banasik JL. *Pathophysiology*, ed 5, St. Louis, 2013, Saunders.)

(25 mm/second × 0.04 second = 1 mm). The rate at which ECG paper goes through the printer is adjustable.

The lines after every five small boxes on the paper are heavier. The heavier lines indicate one large box. Because each large box is the width of five small boxes, a large box represents 0.20 second. Five large boxes, each consisting of five small boxes, represent 1 second; 15 large boxes equal an interval of 3 seconds; and 30 large boxes represent 6 seconds.

The vertical axis of the graph paper represents the voltage or amplitude of the ECG waveforms or deflections. Voltage is measured in millivolts (mV). Voltage may appear as a positive or negative value because voltage is a force with direction and amplitude. Amplitude is measured in millimeters (mm). The default value for ECG machine calibration is 10 mm/mV, which means that when the ECG machine is calibrated correctly, a 1-mV electrical signal produces a deflection that measures precisely 10 mm tall (i.e., the height of 10 small boxes). Clinically, the height of a waveform is usually stated in mm rather than in mV.

WAVEFORMS

A *waveform* (i.e., a deflection) is movement away from the baseline in a positive (i.e., upward) or negative (i.e., downward) direction. Each waveform seen on an ECG is related to a specific electrical event in the heart. Waveforms are named alphabetically, beginning with P, QRS, T, and occasionally U. When electrical activity is not detected, a straight line is recorded. This line is called the *baseline* or *isoelectric line*.

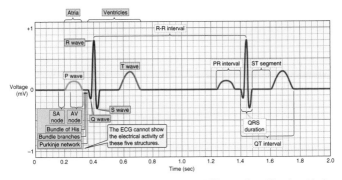

Fig. 2.10 Components of the electrocardiogram (ECG) recording. *AV*, atrioventricular; *SA*, sinoatrial. (From Boron WF, Boulpaep EL. *Medical physiology*, ed 3, Philadelphia, 2017, Elsevier.)

P Wave

The first waveform in the cardiac cycle is the P wave (Fig. 2.10). The P wave represents the spread of the electrical impulse throughout the right and left atria (i.e., atrial depolarization). A P wave normally precedes each QRS complex. The beginning of the P wave is recognized as the first abrupt or gradual movement away from the baseline; its end is the point at which the waveform returns to the baseline.

QRS Complex

A *complex* consists of several waveforms. The QRS complex consists of the Q wave, R wave, and S wave (see Fig. 2.10) and represents the spread of the electrical impulse through the ventricles (i.e., ventricular depolarization) and the sum of all ventricular muscle cell depolarizations. Ventricular depolarization normally triggers the contraction of ventricular tissue. Thus, shortly after the QRS complex begins, the ventricles contract.

A QRS complex normally follows each P wave. One or even two of the three waveforms that make up the QRS complex may not always be present. When it is present, the Q wave is the first downward deflection following the P wave, and it represents depolarization of the interventricular septum. A Q wave is *always* a negative waveform. The Q wave begins when it leaves the isoelectric line in a downward direction and continues until it returns to the isoelectric line. The R wave is the first positive (i.e., upright) waveform following the P wave. The S wave is the negative waveform following the R wave. An R wave is *always* positive, and an S wave is *always* negative. The R and S waves represent depolarization of the right and left ventricles.

The QRS duration is a measurement of the time required for ventricular depolarization. A QRS complex's width is most accurately determined when it is viewed and measured in more than one lead. The measurement should be taken from the QRS complex with the longest duration and clearest onset and end. The beginning of the QRS complex is measured from the point where the first wave of the complex begins to deviate from the baseline. The point at which the last wave of the complex begins to level out or distinctly change direction at, above, or below the baseline marks the QRS complex's end. In adults, the normal duration of the QRS complex is 0.11 second or less (Bagliani et al., 2019; Surawicz et al., 2009). If an electrical impulse does not follow the normal ventricular conduction pathway, it will take longer to depolarize the myocardium. This delay in conduction through the ventricle produces a wider QRS complex.

T Wave

The T wave represents the repolarization of both ventricles. The normal T wave is slightly asymmetric: The waveform's peak is closer to its end than the beginning, and the first half has a more gradual slope than the second half. The beginning of the T wave is identified as the point where the ST segment's slope appears to become abruptly or gradually steeper. The T wave ends when it returns to the baseline. The T-wave direction is usually the same as the QRS complex that precedes it.

U Wave

A U wave is a small waveform that, when seen, follows the T wave. The U wave is thought to represent the late repolarization of the Purkinje fibers (Lederer, 2017). However, some cardiologists believe that U waves are simply two-part T waves resulting from a longer action potential duration in some ventricular myocardial cells (Patton & Thibodeau, 2019). U waves are most easily seen when the heart rate is slow and are difficult to identify when the rate exceeds 95 beats/min (Rautaharju et al., 2009). U waves usually appear in the same direction as the T waves that precede them.

SEGMENTS

A *segment* is a line between waveforms. It is named by the waveform that precedes or follows it.

PR Segment

The PR segment is part of the PR interval (see below), specifically, the horizontal line between the end of the P wave and the beginning of the QRS complex (Fig. 2.11). The PR segment usually is isoelectric and represents the spread of the electrical impulse from the AV node, through the AV bundle, the right and left bundle branches, and the Purkinje fibers to activate ventricular muscle.

TP Segment

The TP segment is the portion of the ECG tracing between the end of the T wave and the beginning of the next P wave, during which there

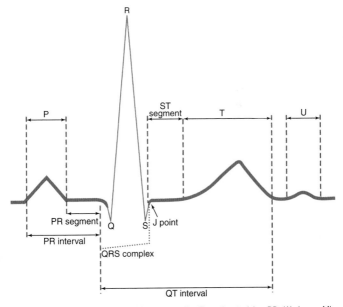

Fig. 2.11 Waveforms, segments, and intervals. (From Ignatavicius DD, Workman ML. *Medical-surgical nursing: patient-centered collaborative care*, 8 ed, St. Louis, 2016, Elsevier.)

is no electrical activity (see Fig. 2.11). When the heart rate is within normal limits, the TP segment is usually isoelectric.

ST Segment

The portion of the ECG tracing between the QRS complex and the T wave is the ST segment. The term ST segment is used regardless of whether the final wave of the QRS complex is an R or an S wave. The ST segment represents the early part of the repolarization of the right and left ventricles. The normal ST segment begins at the isoelectric line, extends from the end of the S wave, and curves gradually upward to the beginning of the T wave.

The junction where the QRS complex and the ST segment meet is called the J point (see Fig. 2.11). Deviation of the ST segment is measured as the number of mm of vertical ST segment displacement (at the J point) from the reference point (Thygesen et al., 2018). Some displacement of the ST segment from the isoelectric line is normal and dependent on age, sex, race, and ECG lead.

INTERVALS

An *interval* is made up of a waveform and a segment.

PR Interval

The P wave plus the PR segment equals the PR interval (PRI); thus, the PRI reflects total supraventricular activity (see Fig. 2.11). The PRI is measured from the point where the P wave leaves the baseline to the beginning of the QRS complex. The PRI changes with heart rate but normally measures 0.12 to 0.20 second in adults. As the heart rate increases, the duration of the PRI shortens. A PRI is considered short if it is less than 0.12 second and long if it is more than 0.20 second.

QT Interval

The QT interval is the period from the beginning of the QRS complex to the end of the T wave. It represents total ventricular activity; this is the time from ventricular depolarization (i.e., activation) to repolarization (i.e., recovery) (see Fig. 2.11). The duration of the QT interval varies with age, sex, and heart rate. As the heart rate increases, the QT interval shortens (i.e., decreases). As the heart rate decreases, the QT interval lengthens (i.e., increases). Generally, a normal QT interval is between 0.40 and 0.44 second. Because of the variability of the QT interval with the heart rate, it can be measured more accurately if corrected (i.e., adjusted) for the patient's heart rate. A corrected QT interval is noted as QTc. In adults, the QTc is considered prolonged if it measures 0.47 second or more in men and 0.48 second or more in women.

R-R and P-P Intervals

The R-R (R wave-to-R wave) and P-P (P wave-to-P wave) intervals are used to determine a cardiac rhythm's rate and regularity. The interval between two consecutive R waves is measured to evaluate the ventricular rhythm's regularity on a rhythm strip (see Fig. 2.10). The distance between succeeding R-R intervals is measured and compared. If the ventricular rhythm is regular, the R-R intervals will measure the same. Atrial regularity is similarly evaluated, except the interval between two consecutive P waves is measured and compared with succeeding P-P intervals.

SYSTEMATIC RHYTHM INTERPRETATION

A systematic approach to rhythm analysis that is consistently applied when analyzing a rhythm strip is essential (Box 2.1). If you do not develop such an approach, you are more likely to miss something important. Begin analyzing the rhythm strip from left to right.

Assess Regularity

The waveforms on an ECG strip are evaluated for regularity by measuring the distance between the P waves and the QRS complexes. To

---

Box 2.1	Systematic Rhythm Interpretation

1. Assess regularity (atrial and ventricular).
2. Assess rate (atrial and ventricular).
3. Identify and examine waveforms.
4. Assess intervals (e.g., PR, QRS, QT) and examine ST segments.
5. Interpret the rhythm and assess its clinical significance.

determine if the ventricular rhythm is regular or irregular, measure the distance between two consecutive R-R intervals. If the ventricular rhythm is regular, the R-R intervals will be equal (measure the same). If the intervals are unequal, the ventricular rhythm is considered irregular. To determine if the atrial rhythm is regular or irregular, follow the same procedure previously described for evaluation of ventricular rhythm but measure the distance between two consecutive P-P intervals (instead of R-R intervals) and compare that distance to the other P-P intervals. The P-P intervals will measure the same if the atrial rhythm is regular. If the intervals are unequal, the atrial rhythm is considered irregular.

Assess Rate

Calculating the heart rate is essential because deviations from normal can affect the patient's ability to maintain an adequate blood pressure and cardiac output. Although the atrial and ventricular rates are usually the same, they differ in some dysrhythmias; therefore, you must calculate both rates. There are several methods used for calculating heart rate. A discussion of each method follows.

Six-Second Method

Most ECG paper is printed with 1-second or 3-second markers on the top or bottom of the paper. On ECG paper, 5 large boxes = 1 second, 15 large boxes = 3 seconds, and 30 large boxes = 6 seconds. To determine the ventricular rate, count the number of complete QRS complexes within 6 seconds, and multiply that number by 10 to find the number of complexes in 1 minute (Fig. 2.12). The 6-second method, also called the

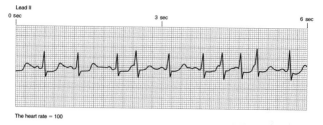

Fig. 2.12 Calculating heart rate using the 6-second method. (From Sole ML, Klein DG, Moseley MJ. *Introduction to critical care nursing*, ed 7, St. Louis, 2017, Elsevier.)

rule of 10, can be used for regular and irregular rhythms. This is the simplest, quickest, and most commonly used method of rate measurement, but it also is the most inaccurate.

Large Box Method

The large box method of rate determination is also called the rule of 300. To determine the ventricular rate, count the number of large boxes between an R-R interval and divide into 300 (Fig. 2.13). Alternately, select an R wave that falls on a dark vertical line. Number the next six consecutive dark vertical lines as follows: 300, 150, 100, 75, 60, and 50 (see Fig. 2.13). Note where the next R wave falls in relation to the six dark vertical lines already marked. This is the heart rate. To determine the atrial rate, count the number of large boxes between a P-P interval and divide into 300 (Table 2.5). This method is best used if the rhythm is regular; however, it may be used if the rhythm is irregular and a rate range (slowest [longest R-R interval] and fastest [shortest R-R interval] rate) is given.

Small Box Method

The small box method of rate determination is also called the rule of 1500. Each 1-mm box on the graph paper represents 0.04 second. A total of 1500 boxes represents 1 minute (60 second/min divided by 0.04 second/box = 1500 boxes/min). To calculate the ventricular rate, count the number of small boxes between an R-R interval and divide

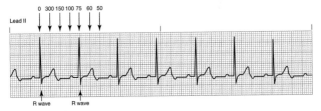

Fig. 2.13 Calculating heart rate using the large box method. To measure the ventricular rate, find an R wave that falls on a heavy dark line. Count the number of large boxes between that R wave and the one that follows it. Divide 300 by the number of large boxes between these R waves. Alternately, using the large boxes, count 300, 150, 100, 75, 60, and 50 until a second R wave occurs. This will be the heart rate. In this example, the second R wave occurs just before the arrow reading a rate of 75 beats/min; thus, the heart rate in this example is about 75 beats/min. (From Sole ML, Klein DG, Moseley MJ. *Introduction to critical care nursing*, ed 7, St. Louis, 2017, Elsevier.)

TABLE 2.5	Heart Rate Determination Based on the Number of Large Boxes	
Number of Large Boxes		**Heart Rate (beats/min)**
1		300
2		150
3		100
4		75
5		60
6		50
7		43
8		38
9		33
10		30

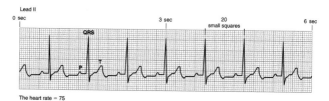

Fig. 2.14 Calculating heart rate using the small box method. To measure the ventricular rate, find an R wave that falls on a heavy dark line. Count the number of small boxes between that R wave and the one that follows it. Divide 1500 by the number of small boxes between these R waves; this will be the heart rate (1500 ÷ 2 = 75 beats/min). (From Sole ML, Klein DG, Moseley MJ. *Introduction to critical care nursing*, ed 7, St. Louis, 2017, Elsevier.)

into 1500 (Fig. 2.14). To determine the atrial rate, count the number of small boxes between a P-P interval and divide into 1500. This method is time-consuming but accurate.

Identify and Examine Waveforms

Look to see if the normal waveforms (P, Q, R, S, and T) are present. To locate P waves, look to the left of each QRS complex. Normally, one P wave precedes each QRS complex; they occur regularly (P-P intervals are equal); and they look similar in size, shape, and position. Next, evaluate the QRS complex. Are QRS complexes present? If so, does a QRS follow each P wave? Do the QRS complexes look alike? Assess the T waves. Does a T wave follow each QRS complex? Does a P wave follow the T wave? Are the T waves upright and of normal height? Look to see if a U wave is present. If so, note its height and direction (positive or negative).

Assess Intervals and Examine Segments

PR Interval

Intervals are measured to evaluate conduction. Is a PRI present? If so, measure the PRIs and determine if they are equal. The PRI is measured from the point at which the P wave leaves the baseline to the beginning of the QRS complex. Are the PRIs within normal limits? Remember that a normal PRI measures 0.12 to 0.20 second. If the PRIs are the same, they are said to be constant. If the PRIs are different, is a pattern present? In some dysrhythmias, the PRI duration gradually increases until a P wave appears with no QRS after it. This pattern is referred to as the lengthening of the PRI. PRIs that vary in duration and have no pattern are said to be variable.

QRS Duration

Identify the QRS complexes and measure their duration. The beginning of the QRS is measured from the point where the first wave of the complex begins to deviate from the baseline. The point at which the last wave of the complex begins to level out at, above, or below the baseline marks the QRS complex's end. The QRS is considered narrow (i.e., normal) if it measures 0.11 second or less and wide if it measures more than 0.11 second. A narrow QRS complex is presumed to be supraventricular in origin.

QT Interval

To determine the QT interval, count the number of small boxes between the beginning of the QRS complex and the end of the T wave. Then multiply that number by 0.04 second. If no Q wave is present, measure the QT interval from the beginning of the R wave to the end of the T wave. The QT interval generally measures 0.40 to 0.44 second. A corrected QT interval (QTc) is considered prolonged in adults if it measures 0.47 second or more in men and 0.48 second or more in women.

Examine ST Segments

Determine the presence of ST-segment elevation or depression. Start by identifying the onset of the QRS, which serves as the reference point. Next, locate the J point and then compare the ST segment level with the reference point. Deviation is measured as the number of mm of vertical ST segment displacement (at the J point) from the reference point.

Interpret the Rhythm

Interpret the rhythm, specifying the site of origin (pacemaker site) of the rhythm (sinus), the mechanism (bradycardia), and the ventricular rate (for example, "Sinus bradycardia at 38 beats/min)." Assess the patient to find out how they are tolerating the rate and rhythm.

REFERENCES

Bagliani, G., Brugada, J., De Ponti, R., Viola, G., Berne, P., & Leonelli, F. M. (2019). QRS variations during arrhythmias: Mechanisms and substrates. Toward a precision electrocardiology. *Card Electrophysiol Clin, 11*(2), 315–331.

Costanzo, L. S. (2018). Cardiovascular physiology. In *Physiology* (6 ed., pp. 117–188). Philadelphia, PA: Elsevier.

Issa, Z. F., Miller, J. M., & Zipes, D. P. (2019). Molecular mechanisms of cardiac electrical activity. In *Clinical arrhythmology and electrophysiology* (3 ed., pp. 1–14). Philadelphia, PA: Elsevier.

Krahn, A. D., Yee, R., Skanes, A. C., & Klein, G. J. (2018). Cardiac monitoring: short- and long-term recording. In D. P. Zipes, J. Jalife, & W. G. Stevenson (Eds.), *Cardiac electrophysiology: From cell to bedside* (7 ed., pp. 623–629). Philadelphia, PA: Elsevier.

Lederer, W. J. (2017). Cardiac electrophysiology and the electrocardiogram. In W. F. Boron & E. L. Boulpaep (Eds.), *Medical physiology* (3 ed., pp. 483–506). Philadelphia, PA: Elsevier.

Pappano, A. J., & Wier, W. G. (2019). Excitation: The cardiac action potential. In *Cardiovascular physiology* (11 ed., pp. 10–28). Philadelphia, PA: Elsevier.

Patton, K. T., & Thibodeau, G. A. (2019). Heart. In *Anatomy & physiology* (10 ed., pp. 634–662). St. Louis, MO: Elsevier.

Peterson, K. (2018). Advanced dysrhythmias. In V. S. Good & P. L. Kirkwood (Eds.), *Advanced critical care nursing* (2 ed., pp. 12–33). St. Louis, MO: Elsevier.

Rautaharju, P. M., Surawicz, B., & Gettes, L. S. (2009). AHA/ACCF/HRS recommendations for the standardization and interpretation of the electrocardiogram: Part IV: the ST segment, T and U waves, and the QT interval. *J Am Coll Cardiol, 53*(11), 982–991.

Shen, W.-K., Sheldon, R. S., Benditt, D. G., Cohen, M. I., Forman, D. E., Goldberger, Z. D., . . . Yancy, C. W. (2017). 2017 ACC/AHA/HRS guideline for the evaluation and management of patients with syncope: a report of the American College of Cardiology/American Heart Association Task Force on Clinical Practice Guidelines and the Heart Rhythm Society. *J Am Coll Cardiol, 70*(5), e39–110.

Surawicz, B., Childers, R., Deal, B. J., & Gettes, L. S. (2009). AHA/ACCF/HRS recommendations for the standardization and interpretation of the electrocardiogram: Part III: intraventricular conduction disturbances: a scientific statement from the American Heart Association Electrocardiography and Arrhythmias Committee. *J Am Coll Cardiol, 53*(11), 976–981.

Thygesen, K., Alpert, J. S., Jaffe, A. S., Chaitman, B. R., Bax, J. J., Morrow, D. A., & White, H. D. (2018). Fourth universal definition of myocardial infarction. *J Am Coll Cardiol, 72*(18), 2231–2264.

Wagner, G. (2012). Basic electrocardiography. In S. Saksena & A. J. Camm (Eds.), *Electrophysiological disorders of the heart* (2 ed., pp. 125–158). Philadelphia, PA: Saunders.

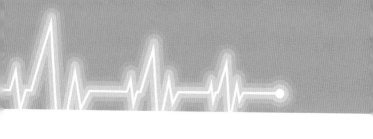

Sinus Mechanisms

3

The normal heartbeat is the result of an electrical impulse that starts in the sinoatrial (SA) node (Fig. 3.1). Normally, pacemaker cells within the SA node spontaneously depolarize more rapidly than other cardiac cells. As a result, the SA node usually dominates other areas that may be depolarizing at a slightly slower rate.

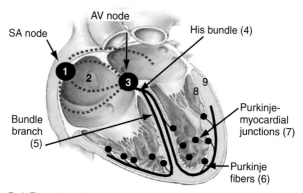

Fig. 3.1 The cardiac action potential originates in the sinoatrial (SA) node (*1*), continues in the atrial wall (*2*), and is delayed in the atrioventricular (AV) node (*3*). Conduction within the ventricles is initially rapid within the rapid conduction system: His bundle (*4*), right and left bundle branches (*5*), and Purkinje fibers (*6*). The impulse is transferred from the rapid conduction system to the working myocardium in the Purkinje-myocardial junctions (*7*) located in the endocardium. Within the slowly conducting working myocardium, the impulse is conducted from endocardium to epicardium. The SA node normally depolarizes faster than any other part of the heart's conduction system. As a result, the SA node usually is the heart's primary pacemaker. (From Ellenbogen KA, Wilkoff BL, Kay GN, Lau CP, Auricchio A. *Clinical cardiac pacing, defibrillation and resynchronization therapy*, ed 5, Philadelphia, 2017, Elsevier.)

A rhythm that begins in the SA node has the following characteristics:

- A positive (i.e., upright) P wave before each QRS complex
- P waves that look alike
- A constant PR interval
- A regular atrial and ventricular rhythm (usually)

SINUS RHYTHM

Sinus rhythm is the name given to a normal heart rhythm. Sinus rhythm is sometimes called a regular sinus rhythm (RSR) or normal sinus rhythm (NSR). Sinus rhythm reflects normal electrical activity—that is, the rhythm starts in the SA node and then heads down the normal conduction pathway through the atria, atrioventricular (AV) node and bundle, right and left bundle branches, and Purkinje fibers. In adults and adolescents, the SA node usually fires at a regular rate of 60 to 100 beats per minute (beats/min). ECG characteristics of a sinus rhythm include the following:

Rhythm:	R-R and P-P intervals are regular
Rate:	60 to 100 beats/min
P waves:	Positive (upright) in lead II; one precedes each QRS complex; P waves look alike
PR interval:	0.12 to 0.20 second and constant from beat to beat
QRS duration:	0.11 second or less unless abnormally conducted

Fig. 3.2 shows an example of a sinus rhythm recorded simultaneously in three leads.

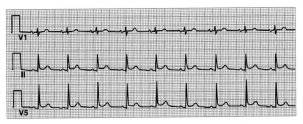

Fig. 3.2 Sinus rhythm at 79 beats/min with ST-segment elevation.

SINUS BRADYCARDIA

If the SA node fires at a rate slower than expected for the patient's age, the rhythm is called *sinus bradycardia*. The rhythm starts in the SA node and then travels the normal conduction pathway, resulting in atrial and ventricular depolarization. In adults and adolescents, sinus bradycardia has a heart rate of less than 60 beats/min. Sinus bradycardia has the following characteristics (Fig. 3.3):

Rhythm:	R-R and P-P intervals are regular
Rate:	Less than 60 beats/min
P waves:	Positive (upright) in lead II; one precedes each QRS complex; P waves look alike
PR interval:	0.12 to 0.20 second and constant from beat to beat
QRS duration:	0.11 second or less unless abnormally conducted

A patient with an unusually slow heart rate may complain of dizziness or lightheadedness, fatigue, weakness, or confusion resulting from decreased cerebral blood flow (Sidhu & Marine, 2020). Decreasing cardiac output will eventually produce hemodynamic compromise. If a patient presents with a bradycardia, assess how they are tolerating the rhythm. If the patient has no symptoms, no treatment is necessary. The term *symptomatic bradycardia* refers to signs and symptoms of hemodynamic compromise related to a slow heart rate. Treatment of symptomatic bradycardia should include assessing the patient's oxygen saturation level and determining if signs of increased breathing effort are present (e.g., retractions, tachypnea). Give supplemental oxygen if oxygenation is inadequate and assist breathing if ventilation is inadequate. Establish intravenous (IV) access and obtain a 12-lead

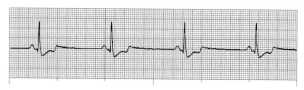

Fig. 3.3 Sinus bradycardia at 40 beats/min with ST-segment depression and inverted T waves.

ECG. Atropine, administered intravenously, is the drug of choice for symptomatic bradycardia. Reassess the patient's response and continue monitoring the patient.

SINUS TACHYCARDIA

If the SA node fires at a rate faster than normal for the patient's age, the rhythm is called *sinus tachycardia*. Sinus tachycardia begins and ends gradually. The rhythm starts in the SA node and travels the normal pathway of conduction through the heart, resulting in atrial and ventricular depolarization. Sinus tachycardia looks much like a sinus rhythm, except that it is faster. It may be hard to tell the difference between a P wave and a T wave at very fast rates. In adults, the ventricular rate associated with sinus tachycardia is faster than 100 beats/min with the maximum rate of about 220 beats/min, minus the patient's age in years. The ventricular rate is usually less than 220 beats/min in infants or 180 beats/min in children. A sinus tachycardia has the following characteristics (Fig. 3.4):

Rhythm:	R-R and P-P intervals are regular
Rate:	Ventricular rate faster than 100 beats/min with the maximum rate about 220 beats/min, minus the patient's age in years
P waves:	Positive (upright) in lead II; one precedes each QRS complex; P waves look alike
PR interval:	0.12 to 0.20 second and constant from beat to beat
QRS duration:	0.11 second or less unless abnormally conducted

Whereas sinus tachycardia is an expected physiologic response to increased oxygen demand, inappropriate sinus tachycardia (IST) describes a sinus tachycardia that occurs for no apparent physiologic

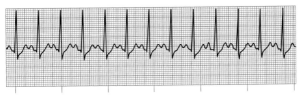

Fig. 3.4 Sinus tachycardia at 125 beats/min with ST-segment depression.

cause. For example, a person's heart rate may rapidly increase to more than 100 beats/min with minimal exertion, at rest, or both. Accompanying symptoms are usually nonspecific and include weakness, dizziness, fatigue, headache, shortness of breath, exercise intolerance, lightheadedness, chest discomfort, a racing heart, or palpitations. The mechanisms responsible for IST are not entirely understood, and a diagnosis is made only after other causes for the tachycardia have been ruled out (Yasin et al., 2018).

Treatment for physiologic sinus tachycardia is directed at correcting the underlying cause (i.e., fluid replacement, relief of pain, removal of offending medications or substances, reducing fever or anxiety). In a patient experiencing an acute myocardial infarction (MI), sinus tachycardia may be treated with medications to slow the heart rate and decrease myocardial oxygen demand (e.g., beta-blockers), provided there are no signs of heart failure or other contraindications.

Treatment of IST can be tricky. Lifestyle modifications are usually recommended. Pharmacologic treatment with beta-blockers or calcium blockers may be tried but is often ineffective, and symptoms can persist despite heart rate control. Ivabradine (Corlanor), a medication usually used to treat heart failure, has proved helpful in treating some IST patients. Surgical ablation may be performed in severe cases.

SINUS ARRHYTHMIA

When the SA node fires irregularly, the resulting rhythm is called *sinus arrhythmia*. Sinus arrhythmia associated with the phases of breathing and changes in intrathoracic pressure is called *respiratory sinus arrhythmia*. Sinus arrhythmia unrelated to the ventilatory cycle is called *nonrespiratory sinus arrhythmia*. ECG characteristics of sinus arrhythmia include the following (Fig. 3.5)

Rhythm:	Irregular and often phasic with breathing; heart rate increases gradually during inspiration (R-R intervals shorten) and decreases with expiration (R-R intervals lengthen)
Rate:	Usually 60 to 100 beats/min
P waves:	Positive (upright) in lead II; one precedes each QRS complex; P waves look alike
PR interval:	0.12 to 0.20 second and constant from beat to beat
QRS duration:	0.11 second or less unless abnormally conducted

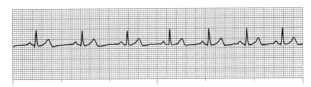

Fig. 3.5 Sinus arrhythmia at 70 beats/min.

Sinus arrhythmia usually does not require treatment unless it is accompanied by a slow heart rate that causes hemodynamic compromise. Intravenous (IV) atropine may be indicated to treat the bradycardia if hemodynamic compromise is present because of the slow rate.

SINOATRIAL BLOCK

With SA block, also called *sinus exit block*, the SA node's pacemaker cells initiate an impulse, but it is blocked as it exits the SA node, resulting in periodically absent PQRST complexes. SA block is thought to occur because of the failure of the transitional cells in the SA node to conduct the impulse from the pacemaker cells to the surrounding atrium. ECG characteristics of SA block include the following (Fig. 3.6):

Rhythm:	Irregular because of the pause(s) caused by the SA block—the pause is the same as, or an exact multiple of, the distance between two other P-P intervals
Rate:	Usually normal but varies because of the pause
P waves:	When present, positive (upright) in lead II; one precedes each QRS complex; P waves look alike
PR interval:	When present, 0.12 to 0.20 second and constant from beat to beat
QRS duration:	0.11 second or less unless abnormally conducted

Signs and symptoms associated with SA block depend on the number of sinus beats blocked. If the SA block episodes are transient and there are no significant signs or symptoms, the patient is observed. If signs of hemodynamic compromise are present and result from medication toxicity, the offending agents should be withheld. If the SA block episodes are frequent, IV atropine, temporary pacing, or insertion of a permanent pacemaker may be needed.

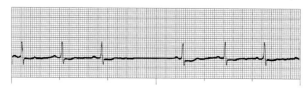

Fig. 3.6 Sinus rhythm at 60 beats/min with an episode of sinoatrial block.

SINUS ARREST

With sinus arrest, the SA node's pacemaker cells do not initiate an electrical impulse for one or more beats resulting in absent PQRST complexes on the ECG.

When the SA node fails to initiate an impulse, an escape pacemaker site (i.e., the AV junction or the Purkinje fibers) should kick in and assume responsibility for pacing the heart. The term *junctional* denotes a beat or rhythm originating at the AV junction. Therefore, when the SA node does not fire and an escape pacemaker kicks in, the pause associated with a sinus arrest may be terminated by a junctional or ventricular escape beat. If an escape pacemaker site does not fire, you will see absent PQRST complexes on the ECG (Fig. 3.7). The following are ECG characteristics of sinus arrest:

Rhythm:	Irregular; the pause is of undetermined length, more than one PQRST complex is missing, and it is not the same distance as other P-P intervals
Rate:	Usually normal but varies because of the pause
P waves:	When present, positive (upright) in lead II; one precedes each QRS complex; P waves look alike
PR interval:	When present, 0.12 to 0.20 second and constant from beat to beat
QRS duration:	0.11 second or less unless abnormally conducted

Signs and symptoms associated with sinus arrest depend on the number of absent sinus beats and the length of the sinus arrest because there is no cardiac output during the period of arrest. If the episodes of sinus arrest are transient and there are no significant signs or symptoms, observe the patient. If hemodynamic compromise is present,

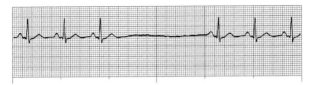

Fig. 3.7 Sinus rhythm at 60 beats/min with an episode of sinus arrest.

IV atropine, temporary pacing, or both may be indicated. If the episodes of sinus arrest are frequent and prolonged or a result of SA node disease, permanent pacemaker insertion is generally warranted.

REFERENCES

Sidhu, S., & Marine, J. E. (2020). Evaluating and managing bradycardia. *Trends Cardiovasc Med, 30*(5), 265–272.

Yasin, O. Z., Vaidya, V. R., Chacko, S. R., & Asirvatham, S. J. (2018). Inappropriate sinus tachycardia: current challenges and future directions. *J Innov Cardiac Rhythm Manage, 9*(7), 3239–3243.

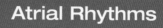

Atrial Rhythms 4

A rhythm that begins in the sinoatrial (SA) node has one positive (i.e., upright) P wave before each QRS complex. A rhythm that begins in the atria will have a positive P wave that is shaped differently than P waves that begin in the SA node. This difference in P wave configuration occurs because the impulse begins in the atria and follows a different conduction pathway to the atrioventricular (AV) node.

PREMATURE ATRIAL COMPLEXES

Premature beats appear early, that is, they occur before the next expected beat. A premature atrial complex (PAC) occurs when an irritable site (i.e., focus) within the atria fires before the next SA node impulse is expected to fire, interrupting the sinus rhythm. If the irritable site is close to the SA node, the atrial P wave will look very similar to the P waves initiated by the SA node. The P wave of a PAC may be biphasic (i.e., partly positive, partly negative), flattened, notched, pointed, or lost in the preceding T wave. ECG characteristics of PACs include the following (Fig. 4.1):

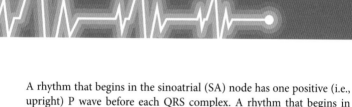

Fig. 4.1 Sinus tachycardia at 111 beasts/min with three premature atrial complexes (PACs). From the left, beats 2, 7, and 10 are PACs.

Rhythm:	Irregular because of the early beat(s)
Rate:	Usually within normal range but depends on underlying rhythm
P waves:	Premature (occurring earlier than the next expected sinus P wave), positive (upright) in lead II, one before each QRS complex, often differ in shape from sinus P waves—may be flattened, notched, pointed, biphasic, or lost in the preceding T wave
PR interval:	May be normal or prolonged depending on the prematurity of the beat
QRS duration:	Usually 0.11 second or less but may be wide (aberrant) or absent, depending on the prematurity of the beat; the QRS of the premature atrial complex (PAC) is similar in shape to those of the underlying rhythm unless the PAC is abnormally conducted

PACs usually do not require treatment if they are infrequent. If PACs are frequent, the patient may notice a skipped beat or occasional palpitations (i.e., the sensation of a racing heart, skipped beats, or flip-flops). Some patients are unaware of their occurrence. In susceptible individuals, frequent PACs may induce episodes of atrial fibrillation (AFib) or paroxysmal supraventricular tachycardia (PSVT). Frequent PACs are treated by correcting the underlying cause.

Noncompensatory versus Compensatory Pause

A noncompensatory (i.e., incomplete) pause often follows a PAC, representing the delay during which the SA node resets its rhythm for the next beat. A compensatory (i.e., complete) pause often follows PVCs (Fig. 4.2). The pause is *noncompensatory* if the period between the complex before and after a premature beat is less than two normal R-R intervals. The pause is *compensatory* if the period between the complex before and after a premature beat is the same as two normal R-R intervals.

Aberrantly Conducted Premature Atrial Complexes

PACs associated with a wide QRS complex are called aberrantly conducted PACs, indicating that conduction through the ventricles

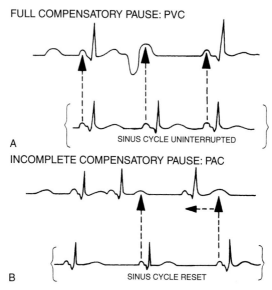

Fig. 4.2 **A**, A full compensatory pause often follows a premature ventricular complex (PVC). **B**, A premature atrial complex (PAC) is often followed by a noncompensatory (incomplete) pause. (From Crawford MV, Spence MI. *Commonsense approach to coronary care*, rev ed 6, St. Louis, 1994, Mosby.)

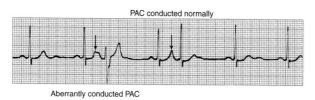

Fig. 4.3 Premature atrial complexes (PACs) with and without abnormal conduction (aberrancy). (From Kinney MP, Packa DR. *Andreoli's comprehensive cardiac care*, ed 8, St. Louis, 1996, Mosby.)

is abnormal. Fig. 4.3 shows a rhythm strip with two PACs. The first PAC (*left arrow*) was conducted abnormally, producing a wide QRS complex. The second PAC (*right arrow*) was conducted normally.

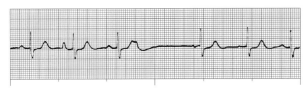

Fig. 4.4 Sinus rhythm with a nonconducted (blocked) premature atrial complex (PAC). Note the distorted T wave of the third QRS complex from the left.

Nonconducted Premature Atrial Complexes

Sometimes when a PAC occurs very early and close to the T wave of the preceding beat, only a P wave may be seen with no QRS after it, appearing as a pause (Fig. 4.4). This type of PAC is called a nonconducted or blocked PAC because the P wave occurred too early to be conducted.

WANDERING ATRIAL PACEMAKER

Multiform atrial rhythm is an updated term for the rhythm formerly known as *wandering atrial pacemaker*. With this rhythm, the P waves' size, shape, and direction vary, sometimes from beat to beat. The difference in the P waves' look results from the gradual shifting of the dominant pacemaker among the SA node, the atria, and/or the AV junction (Fig. 4.5). Wandering atrial pacemaker requires at least three different P waves, seen in the same lead, for proper diagnosis. ECG characteristics of wandering atrial pacemaker include the following:

Rhythm:	Usually irregular as the pacemaker site shifts from the SA node to ectopic atrial locations or AV junction
Rate:	Usually 60 to 100 beats/min but may be slower; if the rate is faster than 100 beats/min, the rhythm is termed multifocal atrial tachycardia
P waves:	Size, shape, and direction may change from beat to beat; may be upright, inverted, biphasic, rounded, flat, pointed, notched, or buried in the QRS complex
PR interval:	Varies as the pacemaker site shifts from the SA node to ectopic atrial locations or AV junction
QRS duration:	0.11 second or less unless abnormally conducted

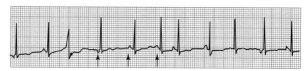

Fig. 4.5 Wandering atrial pacemaker. Note the differences in the shapes of the P waves. (From Paul S, Hebra JD. *The nurse's guide to cardiac rhythm interpretation: Implications for patient care,* Philadelphia, 1998, Saunders.)

Wandering atrial pacemaker is usually a transient rhythm that resolves on its own when the firing rate of the SA node increases and the sinus resumes pacing responsibility.

MULTIFOCAL ATRIAL TACHYCARDIA

When the wandering atrial pacemaker rhythm is associated with a ventricular rate of more than 100 beats/min, the dysrhythmia is called *multifocal atrial tachycardia* (MAT) (Fig. 4.6). As evidenced by its name, MAT results from the random and chaotic firing of multiple ectopic sites in the atria. ECG characteristics of MAT include the following:

Rhythm:	Ventricular rhythm is always irregular as the pacemaker site shifts from the SA node to ectopic atrial locations or AV junction
Rate:	Faster than 100 beats/min
P waves:	One P wave before each QRS but the size, shape, and direction of the P wave may change from beat to beat; may be upright, inverted, biphasic, rounded, flat, pointed, notched, or buried in the QRS complex; at least three different P-wave configurations (seen in the same lead) are required for a diagnosis of multifocal atrial tachycardia.
PR interval:	Varies as the pacemaker site shifts from the SA node to ectopic atrial locations or the AV junction
QRS duration:	0.11 second or less unless abnormally conducted

Because MAT is challenging to treat, it is best to consult a cardiologist before starting treatment. Efforts are focused on managing the underlying cause.

Multifocal Atrial Tachycardia

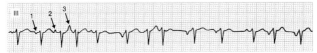

Fig. 4.6 Multifocal atrial tachycardia (MAT). (From Goldberger AL, Goldberger ZD, & Shvilkin A. *Goldberger's clinical electrocardiography: A simplified approach*, ed 9, Philadelphia, 2018, Elsevier.)

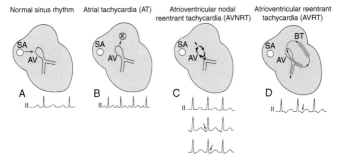

Fig. 4.7 Types of supraventricular tachycardias. **A,** Normal sinus rhythm is shown here as a reference. **B,** With atrial tachycardia (*AT*), a focus (*X*) outside the sinoatrial (*SA*) node fires off automatically at a rapid rate. **C,** With atrioventricular nodal reentrant tachycardia (*AVNRT*), the cardiac stimulus originates as a wave of excitation that spins around the atrioventricular (*AV*) junctional area. As a result, P waves may be buried in the QRS or appear immediately before or just after the QRS complex (*arrows*) because of nearly simultaneous activation of the atria and ventricles. **D,** A similar type of reentrant (circus movement) mechanism in Wolff–Parkinson–White syndrome. This mechanism is referred to as *atrioventricular reentrant tachycardia* (*AVRT*). Note the P wave in lead II somewhat after the QRS complex. *BT,* bypass tract. (From Goldberger AL, Goldberger ZD, & Shvilkin A. *Goldberger's clinical electrocardiography: A simplified approach*, ed 9, Philadelphia, 2018, Elsevier.)

SUPRAVENTRICULAR TACHYCARDIA

Supraventricular arrhythmias begin above the bundle of His; this means that supraventricular arrhythmias include rhythms that begin in the SA node, atrial tissue, or the AV junction. The term supraventricular tachycardia (SVT) includes supraventricular rhythms with a ventricular rate faster than 100 beats/min at rest (Page et al., 2016). Three examples of SVTs are shown above in Fig. 4.7. Sinus tachycardia, which is technically an SVT, is not shown.

Atrial Tachycardia

Atrial tachycardia (AT) is a regular rhythm that arises from an ectopic focus in the atria at a rate faster than 100 beats/min and does not require the AV node's participation to maintain the dysrhythmia (Ellenbogen & Koneru, 2018) (Fig. 4.8). This rapid atrial rate overrides the SA node and becomes the pacemaker. ECG characteristics of AT include the following:

Rhythm:	Regular
Rate:	101 to 250 beats/min
P waves:	One P wave precedes each QRS complex in lead II; these P waves differ in shape from sinus P waves; an isoelectric baseline is usually present between P waves; if the atrial rhythm originates in the low portion of the atrium, P waves will be negative in the inferior leads; with rapid rates, it may be challenging to distinguish P waves from T waves
PR interval:	May be shorter or longer than normal; may be difficult to measure because P waves may be hidden in the T waves of preceding beats
QRS duration:	0.11 second or less unless abnormally conducted

Paroxysmal supraventricular tachycardia (PSVT) is a term used to describe a rapid, regular SVT that starts and ends suddenly. These features are characteristic of atrioventricular nodal reentrant tachycardia (AVNRT) or atrioventricular reentrant tachycardia (AVRT), and, less

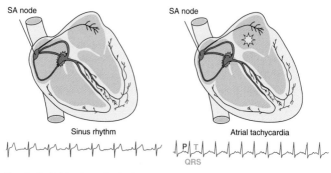

Fig. 4.8 Atrial tachycardia. *SA,* Sinoatrial.

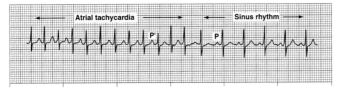

Fig. 4.9 Atrial tachycardia (AT) (a type of supraventricular tachycardia) that ends spontaneously with the abrupt resumption of sinus rhythm. AT that starts or ends suddenly is called *paroxysmal supraventricular tachycardia* (PSVT). The P′ waves of the tachycardia (rate: about 150 beats/min) are superimposed on the preceding T waves. (From Goldberger AL, Goldberger ZD, & Shvilkin A. *Goldberger's clinical electrocardiography: A simplified approach*, ed 9, Philadelphia, 2018, Elsevier.)

frequently, AT (Page et al., 2016) (Fig. 4.9). PSVT may last for minutes, hours, or days. If the onset or end of PSVT is not observed on the ECG, the dysrhythmia is simply called *SVT*.

A rhythm that lasts from 3 beats up to 30 seconds is a *nonsustained rhythm*. A *sustained rhythm* lasts more than 30 seconds or requires pharmacologic or electrical intervention to terminate the rhythm because of hemodynamic instability.

If AT is sustained and the patient is symptomatic because of the rapid rate, treatment should include applying a pulse oximeter and administering oxygen (if indicated), obtaining the patient's vital signs, and establishing IV access. A 12-lead ECG should be obtained. If the patient is not hypotensive, vagal maneuvers may be tried. Although vagal maneuvers are rarely successful, they may be attempted to terminate the rhythm or slow conduction through the AV node. If vagal maneuvers fail, antiarrhythmic medications should be tried if the patient is hemodynamically stable. Adenosine can help restore sinus rhythm or diagnose the tachycardia mechanism in patients with suspected focal AT (Page et al., 2016).

Beta-blockers or calcium blockers may be ordered to slow the ventricular rate (Page et al., 2016). If AT is sustained and causing persistent signs of hemodynamic compromise, IV adenosine may be ordered and, if it is ineffective or if administration is not feasible, synchronized cardioversion should be performed (Page et al., 2016).

Atrioventricular Nodal Reentrant Tachycardia

AVNRT is the most common type of SVT. It results from a reentry circuit that uses two separate pathways leading into the AV node

(Peterson, 2018). One pathway conducts impulses rapidly but has a long refractory period (i.e., slow recovery time). The other pathway conducts impulses slowly but has a short refractory period (i.e., fast recovery time). The pathways join into a final common pathway before impulses exit the AV node and continue to the bundle of His. Under the right conditions, these fast and slow pathways can form an electrical circuit or loop (i.e., a reentry circuit). As one side of the loop is recovering, the other is firing. AVNRT has the following ECG characteristics (Fig. 4.10):

Rhythm:	Ventricular rhythm is usually very regular
Rate:	150 to 250 beats/min
P waves:	Often hidden in the QRS complex; if the ventricles are stimulated first and then the atria, a negative P wave will appear after the QRS in leads II, III, and aVF; when the atria are depolarized after the ventricles, the P wave typically distorts the end of the QRS complex
PR interval:	P waves are not seen before the QRS complex; therefore, the PR interval is not measurable
QRS duration:	0.11 second or less unless abnormally conducted

Because AVNRT may be short-lived or sustained, treatment depends on the tachycardia's duration and severity of the patient's signs and symptoms. If the patient is stable but symptomatic and the symptoms result from the rapid heart rate, apply a pulse oximeter and administer supplemental oxygen, if indicated. Obtain the patient's vital signs, establish IV access, and obtain a 12-lead ECG. While continuously monitoring the patient's ECG, attempt a vagal maneuver if there are no contraindications. If vagal maneuvers do not slow the rate or cause conversion of the tachycardia to a sinus rhythm, the first antiarrhythmic given is adenosine. If the patient is unstable, treatment should include

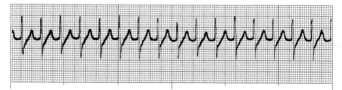

Fig. 4.10 Atrioventricular nodal reentrant tachycardia.

applying a pulse oximeter and administering supplemental oxygen (if indicated), IV access, and sedation (if the patient is awake and time permits) followed by synchronized cardioversion.

Recurrent AVNRT may require treatment with antiarrhythmics. Catheter ablation has become the treatment of choice in managing patients with symptomatic recurrent episodes of AVNRT.

Atrioventricular Reentrant Tachycardia

Preexcitation refers to the premature activation of the ventricles by a supraventricular impulse arising from an accessory pathway. As a result, the impulse excites the ventricles earlier than would be expected if the impulse had traveled through the normal conduction system.

In patients with AVRT, a reentry circuit is formed that often involves four components—the atrium, the normal AV node, the ventricle, and an accessory pathway, also called a bypass tract (Saksena et al., 2012) (Fig. 4.11). Some people have more than one accessory pathway, and several types of accessory pathways have been described. The accessory

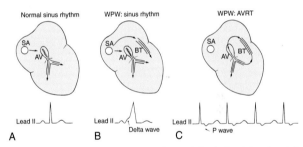

Fig. 4.11 Normal and abnormal conduction pathways. **A,** Conduction during sinus rhythm in the normal heart spreads from the sinoatrial (*SA*) node to the atrioventricular (*AV*) node and then down the bundle branches. The *jagged line* indicates physiologic slowing of conduction in the AV node. **B,** With Wolff–Parkinson–White (*WPW*) pattern, an abnormal accessory conduction pathway called a bypass tract (*BT*) connects the atria and ventricles. With WPW, during sinus rhythm, the electrical impulse is conducted quickly down the bypass tract, preexciting the ventricles before the impulse arrives via the AV node. Consequently, the PR interval is short, and the QRS complex is wide, with slurring at its onset (delta wave). **C,** WPW predisposes patients to develop an atrioventricular reentrant tachycardia (*AVRT*), in which a premature atrial beat may spread down the normal pathway to the ventricles, travel back up the bypass tract, and recirculate down the AV node again. This reentrant loop can repeat itself over and over, resulting in a tachycardia. Notice the normal QRS complex and often negative P wave in lead II during this type of tachycardia. (From Goldberger AL, Goldberger ZD, & Shvilkin A. *Goldberger's clinical electrocardiography: A simplified approach*, ed 9, Philadelphia, 2018, Elsevier.)

pathway's location and the conductive properties of the pathway and AV node determine the extent of preexcitation. Unlike the AV node, an accessory pathway cannot slow or reduce the number of atrial impulses transmitted to the ventricles; therefore, patients with preexcitation syndromes are prone to tachydysrhythmias.

The most common form of preexcitation is the Wolff–Parkinson–White (WPW) pattern. This pattern includes a triad of findings that consists of the following: (1) a short PR interval, (2) a wide QRS complex, and (3) a delta wave (Fig. 4.12). A delta wave is an initial slurred deflection at the beginning of the QRS complex that may be positive or negative. It reflects the relatively slow ventricular depolarization over the accessory pathway (Mark et al., 2009). A patient is said to have a Wolff–Parkinson–White *syndrome* when a WPW preexcitation pattern is present on the ECG, and a tachydysrhythmia occurs that is related to the accessory pathway (Virani et al., 2021). ECG characteristics of the WPW pattern include the following:

Rhythm:	Regular, unless associated with AFib
Rate:	Usually 60 to 100 beats/min if the underlying rhythm is sinus in origin
P waves:	Normal and positive in lead II unless WPW is associated with AFib
PR interval:	0.12 second or less if P waves are observed because the impulse travels very quickly across the accessory pathway, bypassing the normal delay in the AV node
QRS duration:	Usually more than 0.12 second; slurred upstroke of the QRS complex (i.e., delta wave) may be seen in one or more leads

The ECG characteristics of WPW described here are usually seen when the patient is *not* experiencing a tachycardia. WPW syndrome usually goes undetected until it manifests in a patient as a tachycardia. Consultation with a cardiologist is recommended when caring for a patient with AVRT.

ATRIAL FLUTTER AND ATRIAL FIBRILLATION

Atrial flutter is a reentrant rhythm in which an irritable site within the atria fires regularly at a very rapid rate (Fig. 4.13). Typical atrial flutter,

Wolff–Parkinson–White preexcitation

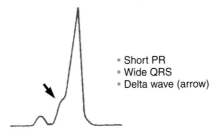

- Short PR
- Wide QRS
- Delta wave (arrow)

Fig. 4.12 Typical Wolff–Parkinson–White (WPW) pattern showing a short PR interval, wide QRS complex and a delta wave. (From Goldberger AL, Goldberger ZD, & Shvilkin A. *Goldberger's clinical electrocardiography: A simplified approach*, ed 9, Philadelphia, 2018, Elsevier).

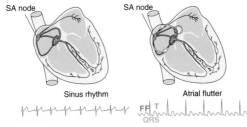

Fig. 4.13 Atrial flutter. *F*, flutter wave.

also known as common atrial flutter, involves a reentry circuit around the right atrium's tricuspid valve. Atrial waveforms are produced that resemble the teeth of a saw or a picket fence; these are called flutter waves or F waves. ECG characteristics of atrial flutter include the following:

Rhythm:	Atrial regular; ventricular regular or irregular depending on AV conduction and blockade
Rate:	Atrial rate typically ranges from 240 to 300 beats/min; ventricular rate varies and is determined by AV blockade; the ventricular rate will usually not exceed 180 beats/min as a result of the intrinsic conduction rate of the AV junction
P waves:	No identifiable P waves; saw-toothed "flutter" waves are present
PR interval:	Not measurable
QRS duration:	0.11 second or less but may be widened if flutter waves are buried in the QRS complex or if abnormally conducted

Atrial fibrillation (AFib) occurs because of altered automaticity in one or several rapidly firing sites in the atria or reentry involving one or more circuits in the atria (Fig. 4.14). Irritable sites in the atria fire at a rate of 300 to 600 times per minute. These rapid impulses cause the muscles of the atria to quiver (i.e., fibrillate), thereby resulting in weak atrial contraction, decreased stroke volume, a subsequent decrease in cardiac output, and a loss of atrial kick. AFib may occur alone or in association with other atrial dysrhythmias. The ECG characteristics of AFib include the following:

Rhythm:	Ventricular rhythm usually irregularly irregular
Rate:	Atrial rate usually 300 to 600 beats/min; ventricular rate variable
P waves:	No identifiable P waves, fibrillatory waves present; erratic, wavy baseline
PR interval:	Not measurable
QRS duration:	0.11 second or less unless abnormally conducted

Treatment decisions for AFib and atrial flutter are based on the ventricular rate, the duration of the rhythm, the patient's general health, and how they tolerate the rhythm. It is best to consult a cardiologist when considering specific therapies. Rate control and rhythm control are the two primary treatment strategies used to control AFib or atrial flutter symptoms. With rate control, the patient remains in atrial flutter or AFib, but the ventricular rate is controlled (i.e., slowed) using medications that prolong the AV node's refractory period (e.g., beta-blockers, calcium blockers) or catheter ablation. With rhythm control, sinus rhythm is reestablished using approaches that may include pharmacologic cardioversion, electric cardioversion, or catheter ablation. Because pharmacologic or electric cardioversion carries a risk of thromboembolism, anticoagulation is recommended before attempting to convert AFib or atrial flutter to a sinus rhythm when the dysrhythmia duration exceeds 48 hours or when the duration is unknown (January et al., 2019).

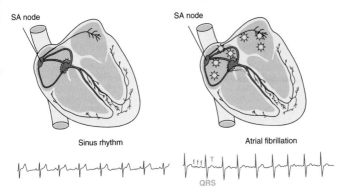

Fig. 4.14 Atrial fibrillation. *f*, fibrillatory wave.

REFERENCES

Ellenbogen, K. A., & Koneru, J. N. (2018). Atrial tachycardia. In D. P. Zipes, J. Jalife, & W. G. Stevenson (Eds.), *Cardiac electrophysiology: From cell to bedside* (7 ed., pp. 681–699). Philadelphia, PA: Elsevier.

January, C. T., Wann, L. S., Calkins, H., Chen, L. Y., Cigarroa, J. E., Cleveland, J. C., & Yancy, C. W. (2019). 2019 AHA/ACC/HRS focused update of the 2014 AHA/ACC/HRS guideline for the management of patients with atrial fibrillation. *Journal of the American College of Cardiology, 74*(1), 104–132.

Mark, D. G., Brady, W. J., & Pines, J. M. (2009). Preexcitation syndromes: Diagnostic consideration in the ED. *Am J Emerg Med, 27*(7), 878–888.

Page, R. L., Joglar, J. A., Caldwell, M. A., Calkins, H., Conti, J. B., Deal, B. J., & Al-Khatib, S. M. (2016). 2015 ACC/AHA/HRS guideline for the management of adult patients with supraventricular tachycardia. *Circulation, 133*(14), e506–e574.

Peterson, K. (2018). Advanced dysrhythmias. In V. S. Good & P. L. Kirkwood (Eds.), *Advanced critical care nursing* (2 ed., pp. 12–33). St. Louis, MO: Elsevier.

Saksena, S., Bharati, S., Lindsay, B. D., & Levy, S. (2012). Paroxysmal supraventricular tachycardia and pre-excitation syndromes. In S. Saksena & A. J. Camm (Eds.), *Electrophysiological disorders of the heart* (2 ed., pp. 531–558). Philadelphia, PA: Saunders.

Virani, S. S., Alonso, A., Aparicio, H. J., Benjamin, E. J., Bittencourt, M. S., Callaway, C. W., & Tsao, C. W. (2021). Heart disease and stroke statistics–2021 update: A report from the American Heart Association. *Circulation, 143*(8), e254–e743.

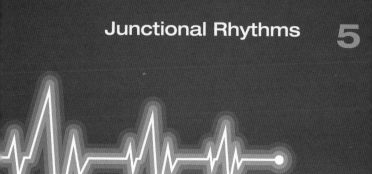

The atrioventricular (AV) node's main job is to delay an electrical impulse, allowing the atria to contract and complete filling of the ventricles with blood before the next ventricular contraction. After passing through the AV node, the electrical impulse enters the bundle of His. The bundle of His, also called the common bundle or the AV bundle, is located in the upper part of the interventricular septum. It connects the AV node with the right and left bundle branches. The bundle of His has pacemaker cells capable of discharging at a rhythmic rate of 40 to 60 beats per minute (beats/min). The AV node and the nonbranching portion of the bundle of His are called the AV junction.

If the AV junction paces the heart, the electrical impulse must travel backward (retrograde) to activate the atria. If a P wave is seen, it will be inverted in leads II, III, and aVF because the impulse is traveling away from the positive electrode (Fig. 5.1). If the atria depolarize before the ventricles, an inverted P wave will be seen *before* the QRS complex, and the PR interval will usually measure 0.12 second or less (Fig. 5.2). The PR interval is shorter than usual because an impulse that begins in the AV junction does not have to travel as far to stimulate the ventricles. If the atria and ventricles depolarize at the same time, a P wave will not be visible because it will be hidden in the QRS complex. When the atria are depolarized after the ventricles, the P wave typically distorts the end of the QRS complex, and an inverted P wave will appear *after* the QRS.

PREMATURE JUNCTIONAL COMPLEXES

A *premature junctional complex* (PJC) occurs when an irritable site within the AV junction fires before the next sinoatrial (SA) node

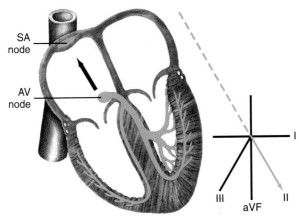

Fig. 5.1 If the atrioventricular (*AV*) junction paces the heart, the electrical impulse must travel in a backward (retrograde) direction to activate the atria. If a P wave is seen, it will be inverted in leads II, III, and aVF because the impulse is traveling away from the positive electrode. *SA*, sinoatrial. (From Grauer K. *A practical guide to ECG* interpretation, ed 2, St. Louis, 1998, Mosby.)

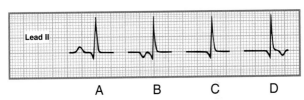

Fig. 5.2 **A**, With a sinus rhythm, the P wave is positive (upright) in lead II because the wave of depolarization is moving toward the positive electrode. The P wave associated with a junctional beat (in lead II) may be inverted (retrograde) and appear before the QRS (**B**), be hidden by the QRS (**C**), or appear after the QRS (**D**). (From Grauer K. *A practical guide to ECG interpretation*, ed 2, St. Louis, 1998, Mosby.)

impulse is ready to fire, interrupting the underlying rhythm. Because the impulse is conducted through the ventricles in the usual manner, the QRS complex will usually measure 0.11 second or less. A PJC is not an entire rhythm; rather, it is a single beat. When identifying a rhythm, be sure to specify the underlying rhythm and the origin of the ectopic beat(s). ECG characteristics of PJCs include the following (Fig. 5.3):

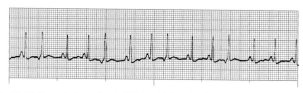

Fig. 5.3 Sinus tachycardia at 140 beats/min with frequent premature junctional complexes.

Rhythm:	Irregular because of the premature beats
Rate:	Usually within normal range but depends on underlying rhythm
P waves:	May occur before, during, or after the QRS; if visible, the P wave is inverted in leads II, III, and aVF
PR interval:	If a P wave occurs before the QRS, the PR interval will usually be 0.12 second or less; if no P wave occurs before the QRS, there will be no PR interval
QRS duration:	0.11 second or less unless abnormally conducted

PJCs do not generally require treatment because most individuals who have PJCs are asymptomatic. However, PJCs may lead to symptoms of palpitations or the feeling of skipped beats. If PJCs occur because of ingestion of stimulants or digitalis toxicity, these substances should be withheld.

JUNCTIONAL ESCAPE BEATS OR RHYTHM

A junctional escape beat begins in the AV junction and appears *late* (i.e., after the next expected beat of the underlying rhythm). ECG characteristics of junctional escape beats include the following (Fig. 5.4):

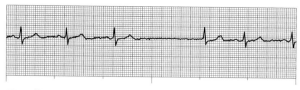

Fig. 5.4 Sinus rhythm at 60 beats/min with an episode of sinus arrest and a junctional escape beat. (From Aehlert B. *ECG study cards*, St. Louis, 2004, Mosby.)

Rhythm:	Irregular because of *late* beats
Rate:	Usually within normal range but depends on underlying rhythm
P waves:	May occur before, during, or after the QRS; if visible, the P wave is inverted in leads II, III, and aVF
PR interval:	If a P wave occurs before the QRS, the PR interval will usually be 0.12 second or less; if no P wave occurs before the QRS, there will be no PR interval
QRS duration:	0.11 second or less unless abnormally conducted

A junctional rhythm is several sequential junctional escape beats. The ECG characteristics of a junctional escape rhythm include the following (Fig. 5.5):

Rhythm:	Very regular
Rate:	40 to 60 beats/min
P waves:	May occur before, during, or after the QRS; if visible, the P wave is inverted in leads II, III, and aVF
PR interval:	If a P wave occurs before the QRS, the PR interval will usually be 0.12 second or less; if no P wave occurs before the QRS, there will be no PR interval
QRS duration:	0.11 second or less unless abnormally conducted

Patients may be asymptomatic with a junctional escape rhythm, or they may experience signs and symptoms associated with the slow heart rate and decreased cardiac output. Treatment depends on the cause of the dysrhythmia, the patient's presenting signs and symptoms, and the frequency and severity of those symptoms. When a patient experiences serious signs and symptoms related to a slow heart rate, treatment should include applying a pulse oximeter, administering supplemental oxygen (if indicated), establishing intravenous (IV) access, and obtaining a 12-lead ECG. Atropine, given IV, is the first medication given for symptomatic bradycardia (Kusumoto et al., 2018). Reassess the patient's response and continue monitoring.

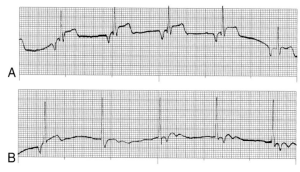

Fig. 5.5 Junctional escape rhythm. Continuous strips. **A,** Note the inverted (retrograde) P waves before the QRS complexes. **B,** Note the change in the location of the P waves. In the first beat, the retrograde P wave is seen before the QRS. In the second beat, no P wave is seen. In the remaining beats, the P wave is seen after the QRS complexes. (From Aehlert B. *ECG study cards*, St. Louis, 2004, Mosby.)

ACCELERATED JUNCTIONAL RHYTHM

If the AV junction speeds up and fires at 61 to 100 beats/min, the resulting rhythm is called an *accelerated junctional rhythm*. ECG characteristics of this rhythm include the following (Fig. 5.6):

Rhythm:	Very regular
Rate:	61 to 100 beats/min
P waves:	May occur before, during, or after the QRS; if visible, the P wave is inverted in leads II, III, and aVF
PR interval:	If a P wave occurs before the QRS, the PR interval will usually be 0.12 second or less; if no P wave occurs before the QRS, there will be no PR interval
QRS duration:	0.11 second or less unless abnormally conducted

The patient is usually asymptomatic because the ventricular rate is 61 to 100 beats/min; however, the patient should be monitored closely. If the patient is symptomatic, treatment is focused on addressing the underlying cause of the dysrhythmia. For example, if the rhythm is caused by digitalis toxicity, this medication should be withheld.

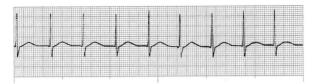

Fig. 5.6 Accelerated junctional rhythm at 93 beats/min.

JUNCTIONAL TACHYCARDIA

Junctional tachycardia is an ectopic rhythm that begins in the pace-maker cells found in the bundle of His. A junctional tachycardia exists when three or more sequential PJCs occur at a rate of more than 100 beats/min. ECG characteristics of junctional tachycardia include the following (Fig. 5.7):

Rhythm:	Ventricular rhythm usually regular, but may be irregular
Rate:	101 to 220 beats/min
P waves:	May occur before, during, or after the QRS; if visible, the P wave is inverted in leads II, III, and aVF
PR interval:	If a P wave occurs before the QRS, the PR interval will usually be 0.12 second or less; if no P wave occurs before the QRS, there will be no PR interval
QRS duration:	0.11 second or less unless abnormally conducted

Junctional tachycardias are usually regular but may be irregular with variable conduction to the atria (Page et al., 2016). *Nonparoxysmal* (i.e., gradual onset) *junctional tachycardia* is a benign dysrhythmia that is usually associated with a gradual increase in rate (i.e., a warm-up pattern) to more than 100 beats/min; it rarely exceeds 120 beats/min (Zimetbaum, 2020). *Paroxysmal junctional tachycardia,* which is also known as *focal* or *automatic junctional tachycardia,* is an uncommon dysrhythmia that starts and ends suddenly and is often precipitated by a PJC. The ventricular rate for paroxysmal junctional tachycardia is generally faster, at a rate of 140 beats/min or more. When the ventricular rate is faster than 150 beats/min, it is challenging to distinguish junctional tachycardia from other supraventricular tachycardias.

Treatment depends on the severity of the patient's signs and symptoms, and expert consultation is advised. If the patient tolerates the rhythm,

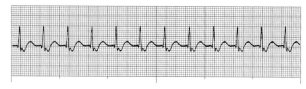

Fig. 5.7 Junctional tachycardia at 115 beats/min.

observation is often all that is needed. If the patient is symptomatic because of the rapid rate, initial treatment should include applying a pulse oximeter, administering supplemental oxygen (if indicated), establishing IV access, and obtaining a 12-lead ECG. Because it is often difficult to distinguish junctional tachycardia from other narrow-QRS tachycardias, vagal maneuvers and, if necessary, IV adenosine may be ordered to help determine the origin of the rhythm. A beta-blocker (e.g., propranolol) or calcium blocker (e.g., diltiazem, verapamil) may be ordered (if no contra-indications exist) to slow conduction through the AV node and thereby slow the ventricular rate. Synchronized cardioversion is not indicated for junctional tachycardia because it typically recurs within seconds after the shock, and a release of endogenous catecholamines following the shock can worsen the dysrhythmia (Miller et al., 2019).

REFERENCES

Kusumoto, F. M., Schoenfeld, M. H., Barrett, C., Edgerton, J. R., Ellenbogen, K. A., Gold, M. R., & Varosy, P. D. (2018). 2018 ACC/AHA/HRS guideline on the evaluation and management of patients with bradycardia and cardiac conduction delay. *Circulation, 140*(8), e382–e482.

Miller, J. M., Tomaselli, G. F., & Zipes, D. P. (2019). Therapy for cardiac arrhythmias. In D. P. Zipes, P. Libby, R. O. Bonow, D. L. Mann, G. F. Tomaselli, & E. Braunwald (Eds.), *Braunwald's heart disease: A textbook of cardiovascular medicine* (11 ed.). Philadelphia, PA: Elsevier.

Page, R. L., Joglar, J. A., Caldwell, M. A., Calkins, H., Conti, J. B., Deal, B. J., . . . Al-Khatib, S. M. (2016). 2015 ACC/AHA/HRS guideline for the management of adult patients with supraventricular tachycardia. *Circulation, 133*(14), e506–e574.

Zimetbaum, P. (2020). Supraventricular cardiac arrhythmias. In L. Goldman & A. I. Schafer (Eds.), *Goldman–Cecil medicine* (26 ed., pp. 331–343). Philadelphia, PA: Elsevier.

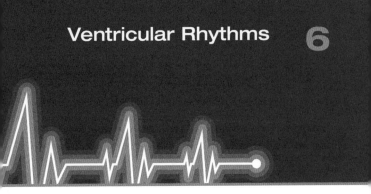

Ventricular Rhythms   6

Ventricular beats and rhythms can start in any part of the ventricles. When an ectopic site within a ventricle assumes responsibility for pacing the heart, the electrical impulse bypasses the normal intraventricular conduction pathway, which results in stimulation of the ventricles at slightly different times. As a result, ventricular beats and rhythms usually have QRS complexes that are abnormally shaped and longer than normal (e.g., greater than 0.11 second). If the atria are depolarized after the ventricles, retrograde P waves may be seen.

Because ventricular depolarization is abnormal, ventricular repolarization is also abnormal and results in ST segment and T wave changes. The T waves are usually in a direction opposite that of the QRS complex; if the major QRS deflection is negative, the ST segment is usually elevated, and the T wave is positive (i.e., upright). If the major QRS deflection is positive, the ST segment is usually depressed, and the T wave is usually negative (i.e., inverted). P waves are usually not seen with ventricular dysrhythmias; however, if they are visible, they have no consistent relationship to the QRS complex.

PREMATURE VENTRICULAR COMPLEXES

A *premature ventricular complex* (PVC) arises from an irritable site within either ventricle. By definition, a PVC is *premature*, occurring earlier than the next expected sinus beat. A compensatory pause often follows a PVC and occurs because the SA node is usually not affected by the PVC. A PVC can occur with any supraventricular dysrhythmia. The general ECG characteristics of PVCs include the following (Fig. 6.1):

Rhythm:	Irregular because of the early beats; if the premature ventricular complex (PVC) is an interpolated PVC, the rhythm will be regular
Rate:	Usually within normal range, but depends on the underlying rhythm
P waves:	Usually absent or, with retrograde conduction to the atria, may appear after the QRS (usually upright in the ST segment or T wave)
PR interval:	None with the PVC because the ectopic beat originates in the ventricles
QRS duration:	Usually 0.12 second or greater; T wave is usually in the opposite direction of the QRS complex

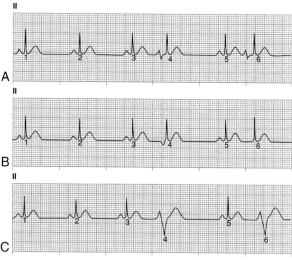

Fig. 6.1 Premature beats. **A,** Sinus rhythm with premature atrial complexes (PACs). The fourth and sixth beats are preceded by premature P waves that look different from the normally conducted sinus beats. Note that the QRS complex that follows each of these PACs is narrow and identical in appearance to that of the sinus-conducted beats. **B,** Sinus rhythm with premature junctional complexes (PJCs). The fourth and sixth beats are PJCs. Beat No. 4 is preceded by an inverted P wave with a short PR interval. There is no identifiable atrial activity associated with beat No. 6. **C,** Sinus rhythm with premature ventricular complexes (PVCs). The fourth and sixth beats are very different in appearance from the normally conducted sinus beats. Beats 4 and 6 are PVCs. P waves do not precede them. (From Grauer K. *A practical guide to ECG interpretation,* ed 2, St. Louis, 1998, Mosby.)

PVCs may occur alone or in groups (i.e., patterns). Frequent PVCs are defined as the presence of at least 1 PVC on a 12-lead ECG or more than 30 PVCs per hour (Al-Khatib et al., 2018). PVCs that infrequently occur with no identifiable pattern are called isolated PVCs. Two consecutive PVCs are called a pair or couplet. Ventricular bigeminy describes a rhythm in which every other beat is a PVC; with ventricular trigeminy, every third beat is a PVC; and with ventricular quadrigeminy, every fourth beat is a PVC.

PVCs that look alike in the same lead and begin from the same anatomic site (i.e., focus) are called uniform PVCs. PVCs that look different from one another in the same lead are called multiform PVCs.

When a PVC occurs between two normally conducted QRS complexes without interfering with the normal cardiac cycle, it is called an interpolated PVC. An R-on-T PVC occurs when the R wave of a PVC falls on the T wave of the preceding beat.

When identifying a patient's cardiac rhythm, first describe the underlying rhythm and then describe the ectopic beats present.

Most patients experiencing PVCs do not require treatment with antiarrhythmic medications; rather, treatment of PVCs focuses on searching for and treating potentially reversible causes. Ambulatory monitoring can help identify the type and frequency of ventricular ectopy.

VENTRICULAR ESCAPE BEATS OR RHYTHM

A ventricular escape beat occurs after a pause in which a supraventricular pacemaker failed to fire; thus, an escape beat is *late*, appearing after the next expected normal beat. A ventricular escape beat is a *protective* mechanism, safeguarding the heart from more extreme slowing or even asystole. The ECG characteristics of ventricular escape beats include the following (Fig. 6.2):

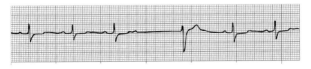

Fig. 6.2 Sinus rhythm with a prolonged PR interval, nonconducted premature atrial complex, ventricular escape beat, and ST-segment depression. (From Chou T, Ramaiah LS. *Electrocardiography in clinical practice: adult and pediatric*, ed 4, Philadelphia, 1996, Saunders.)

Rhythm:	Irregular because of *late* beats; the ventricular escape beat occurs *after* the next expected beat of the underlying rhythm
Rate:	Usually within normal range, but depends on the underlying rhythm
P waves:	Usually absent or, with retrograde conduction to the atria, may appear after the QRS (usually upright in the ST segment or T wave)
PR interval:	None with the ventricular escape beat because the ectopic beat originates in the ventricles
QRS duration:	0.12 second or greater; the T wave is frequently in the opposite direction of the QRS complex

An *idioventricular rhythm (IVR)*, also known as a *ventricular escape rhythm*, exists when three or more ventricular escape beats occur in a row at a rate of 20 to 40 beats/min. When the ventricular rate slows to less than 20 beats/min, some practitioners refer to the rhythm as an agonal rhythm or dying heart. Characteristics of IVR include the following (Fig. 6.3):

Rhythm:	Ventricular rhythm is essentially regular
Rate:	Ventricular rate 20 to 40 beats/min
P waves:	Usually absent or, with retrograde conduction to the atria, may appear after the QRS (usually upright in the ST segment or T wave)
PR interval:	None
QRS duration:	0.12 second or greater; the T wave is frequently in the opposite direction of the QRS complex

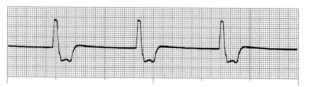

Fig. 6.3 Idioventricular rhythm. (From Aehlert B. *ECG study cards*, St. Louis, 2004, Mosby.)

If the patient has a pulse and is symptomatic because of the slow rate, apply a pulse oximeter and administer supplemental oxygen if indicated. Establish intravenous (IV) access and obtain a 12-lead ECG. Atropine may be ordered to treat the symptomatic bradycardia. If atropine is administered, reassess the patient's response and continue monitoring. Transcutaneous pacing or a dopamine or epinephrine IV infusion may be ordered if atropine is ineffective.

If the patient is not breathing and has no pulse despite the appearance of organized electrical activity on the cardiac monitor, pulseless electrical activity (PEA) exists. Therapeutic interventions for PEA include performing cardiopulmonary resuscitation (CPR), giving oxygen, starting an IV infusion, administering epinephrine, possibly placing an advanced airway, and aggressively searching for the underlying cause.

ACCELERATED IDIOVENTRICULAR RHYTHM

An *accelerated idioventricular rhythm* (AIVR) exists when three or more ventricular beats occur in a row at a rate of 41 to 100 beats/min. The ECG characteristics of AIVR include the following (Fig. 6.4):

Rhythm:	Ventricular rhythm is essentially regular
Rate:	41 to 100 (41 to 120 per some cardiologists) beats/min
P waves:	Usually absent or, with retrograde conduction to the atria, may appear after the QRS (usually upright in the ST segment or T wave)
PR interval:	None
QRS duration:	0.12 second or greater; the T wave is frequently in the opposite direction of the QRS complex

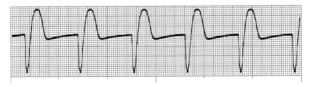

Fig. 6.4 Accelerated idioventricular rhythm. (From Aehlert B. *ECG study cards*, St. Louis, 2004, Mosby.)

AIVR is usually considered a benign escape rhythm. It appears when the sinus rate slows and disappears when the sinus rate speeds up. AIVR generally requires no treatment because the rhythm is protective and often transient, spontaneously resolving on its own.

VENTRICULAR TACHYCARDIA

Ventricular tachycardia (VT) exists when three or more sequential PVCs occur at a rate of more than 100 beats/min. VT may occur with or without pulses, and the patient may be stable or unstable with this rhythm.

VT may occur as a short run that lasts less than 30 seconds and spontaneously ends (i.e., nonsustained VT). Sustained VT persists for more than 30 seconds or requires termination because of resulting hemodynamic compromise in less than 30 seconds (Al-Khatib et al., 2018).

Monomorphic Ventricular Tachycardia

Similar to PVCs, VT may originate from an ectopic focus in either ventricle. When the QRS complexes of VT are of the same shape and amplitude, the rhythm is called monomorphic VT (Fig. 6.5). The ECG characteristics of monomorphic VT include the following:

Rhythm:	Ventricular rhythm is essentially regular
Rate:	101 to 250 (121 to 250 per some cardiologists) beats/min
P waves:	Usually not seen; if present, they have no set relationship with the QRS complexes that appear between them at a rate different from that of the VT
PR interval:	None
QRS duration:	0.12 second or greater; often difficult to differentiate between the QRS and T wave

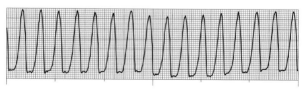

Fig. 6.5 Monomorphic ventricular tachycardia. (From Aehlert B. *ECG study cards*, St. Louis, 2004, Mosby.)

Treatment is based on the patient's signs and symptoms and the type of VT. If the rhythm is monomorphic VT (and the tachycardia is the cause of the patient's symptoms):

- CPR and defibrillation are used to treat the pulseless patient with VT.
- Stable but symptomatic patients are treated with oxygen (if indicated), IV access, and ventricular antiarrhythmics (e.g., procainamide, amiodarone, sotalol) to suppress the rhythm.
- Unstable patients (usually a sustained heart rate of 150 beats/min or more) are treated with oxygen, IV access, and sedation (if the patient is awake and time permits) followed by synchronized cardioversion.

Polymorphic Ventricular Tachycardia

With polymorphic ventricular tachycardia (PMVT), the QRS complexes vary in shape and amplitude from beat to beat and appear to twist from upright to negative or negative to upright and back, resembling a spindle. PMVT is a dysrhythmia of intermediate severity between monomorphic VT and ventricular fibrillation (VF) (Fig. 6.6). It may be challenging to distinguish PMVT from VF when the rate of PMVT is very fast (Garan, 2020). The ECG characteristics of PMVT include the following:

Rhythm:	Ventricular rhythm may be regular or irregular
Rate:	Ventricular rate 150 to 300 beats/min; typically 200 to 250 beats/min
P waves:	None
PR interval:	None
QRS duration:	0.12 second or more; there is a gradual alteration in the amplitude and direction of the QRS complexes; a typical cycle consists of 5 to 20 QRS complexes

Several types of PMVT and their possible causes have been identified. Most PMVTs are associated with a normal QT interval (Jebberi et al., 2019) and are simply referred to as normal-QT PMVT. PMVT that occurs in the presence of a long QT interval (typically 0.45 second or more and often 0.50 second or more) is called *torsades de pointes* (TdP).

It is best to consult a cardiologist when treating a patient with PMVT because of the diverse mechanisms of PMVT, as there may or may not

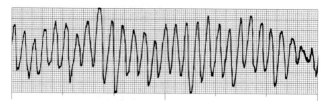

Fig. 6.6 Polymorphic ventricular tachycardia. This rhythm strip is from a 77-year-old man three days after myocardial infarction (MI). His chief complaint at the onset of this episode was chest pain. He had a past medical history of a previous MI and an abdominal aortic aneurysm repair. The patient was given a ventricular antiarrhythmic and defibrillated several times without success. Laboratory work revealed a serum potassium (K⁺) level of 2.0. Intravenous K⁺ was administered, and the patient converted to a sinus rhythm with the next defibrillation.

be clues as to its specific cause at the time of the patient's presentation. Treatment options vary and can be contradictory. For example, a medication that may be appropriate for treating a patient with TdP may be contraindicated when treating a patient with another form of PMVT. In general, if the patient is symptomatic because of the tachycardia, treat ischemia (if it is present), correct electrolyte abnormalities, and discontinue any medications that the patient may be taking that prolong the QT interval.

VENTRICULAR FIBRILLATION

In ventricular fibrillation (VF), the ventricular muscle quivers, and as a result, there is no effective myocardial contraction and no pulse. The resulting rhythm looks chaotic with deflections that vary in shape and amplitude. VF with waves that are 3 or more mm high is called coarse VF. VF with low amplitude waves (i.e., less than 3 mm) is called fine VF. In general, coarse VF is more likely to respond to defibrillation than fine VF. The ECG characteristics of VF include the following (Fig. 6.7):

Rhythm:	Rapid and chaotic with no pattern or regularity
Rate:	Cannot be determined because there are no discernible waves or complexes to measure
P waves:	None
PR interval:	None
QRS duration:	None

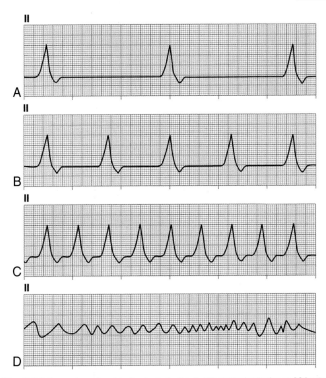

Fig. 6.7 Comparison of ventricular dysrhythmias. **A,** Idioventricular rhythm at 38 beats/min. **B,** Accelerated idioventricular rhythm at 75 beats/min. **C,** Monomorphic ventricular tachycardia at 150 beats/min. **D,** Coarse ventricular fibrillation. (From Grauer K. *A practical guide to ECG interpretation*, ed 2, St. Louis, 1998, Mosby.)

The priorities of care in cardiac arrest resulting from pulseless VT or VF are high-quality CPR and defibrillation. Administer medications and perform additional interventions per current resuscitation guidelines.

ASYSTOLE

Asystole, also called *cardiac standstill*, is a total absence of atrial and ventricular electrical activity (Fig. 6.8). There is no atrial or ventricular rate or rhythm, no pulse, and no cardiac output. If atrial electrical

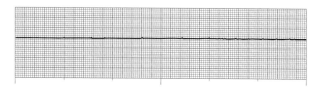

Fig. 6.8 Asystole.

activity is present, the rhythm is called P wave asystole or ventricular standstill. The ECG characteristics of asystole include the following:

Rhythm:	Ventricular not discernible; atrial may be discernible
Rate:	Ventricular not discernible, but atrial activity may be observed (i.e., P wave asystole)
P waves:	Usually none
PR interval:	None
QRS duration:	Absent

When asystole is observed on a cardiac monitor, quickly confirm that the patient is unresponsive and has no pulse, and then begin high-quality CPR. Additional care includes establishing vascular access, considering possible reversible causes of the arrest, administering medications (i.e., epinephrine), and performing additional interventions per current resuscitation guidelines.

REFERENCES

Al-Khatib, S. M., Stevenson, W. G., Ackerman, M. J., Bryant, W. J., Callans, D. J., Curtis, A. B., . . . Page, R. L. (2018). 2017 AHA/ACC/HRS guideline for management of patients with ventricular arrhythmias and the prevention of sudden cardiac death. *Journal of the American College of Cardiology, 72*(14), e91–e220.

Garan, H. (2020). Ventricular arrhythmias. In L. Goldman & A. I. Schafer (Eds.), *Goldman–Cecil medicine* (26 ed., pp. 343–350). Philadelphia, PA: Elsevier.

Jebberi, Z., Marazzato, J., De Ponti, R., Bagliani, G., Leonelli, F. M., & Boveda, S. (2019). Polymorphic wide QRS complex tachycardia: Differential diagnosis. *Card Electrophysiol Clin, 11*(2), 333–344.

INTRODUCTION

When impulse conduction from the atria to the ventricles is delayed or interrupted because of a transient or permanent anatomic or functional impairment in the conduction system, the resulting dysrhythmia is called an *atrioventricular (AV) block* (Issa et al., 2019). When analyzing a rhythm strip, you can assess PR intervals to detect AV conduction disturbances.

AV block is classified into (1) first-degree AV block, (2) second-degree AV block (types I and II), and (3) third-degree AV block. With first-degree AV block, impulses from the SA node to the ventricles are *delayed*; they are not blocked. With second-degree AV blocks, there is an *intermittent* disturbance in the conduction of impulses between the atria and the ventricles. There is a *complete* block in the conduction of impulses between the atria and the ventricles with a third-degree AV block.

First-degree AV block usually occurs because of a conduction delay within the AV node. Second- and third-degree AV blocks can occur at the level of the AV node, within the bundle of His, or below the bundle of His within the bundle branches. AV blocks located at the bundle of His or bundle branches are called infranodal or subnodal AV blocks.

FIRST-DEGREE ATRIOVENTRICULAR BLOCK

With a first-degree AV block, all components of the cardiac cycle are usually within normal limits, except for the PR interval. The PR interval is abnormal because electrical impulses travel in their usual manner from the SA node through the atria but then encounter a delay in impulse conduction, usually at the level of the AV node. Despite its name, the SA node impulse is not blocked during a first-degree AV block; instead, each sinus impulse is *delayed* for the same period before it is conducted to the ventricles. The terms AV delay and delayed AV conduction have been suggested as alternative names for first-degree AV block. Delayed AV conduction results in a PR interval that is longer than normal (i.e., more than 0.20 second in duration in adults) and constant before each QRS complex. The electrocardiogram (ECG) characteristics of first-degree AV block include the following (Fig. 7.1):

Rhythm:	Regular
Rate:	Usually within normal range, but depends on underlying rhythm
P waves:	Normal in size and shape; one positive (upright) P wave before each QRS
PR interval:	Prolonged (i.e., more than 0.20 second) but constant
QRS duration:	Usually 0.11 second or less unless abnormally conducted

Patients with first-degree AV block are often asymptomatic. First-degree AV block that occurs with acute myocardial infarction (MI) should be monitored closely to detect progression to higher-degree AV block. If first-degree AV block accompanies symptomatic bradycardia, treat the bradycardia.

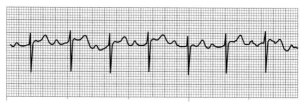

Fig. 7.1 Sinus rhythm at 88 beats/min with a first-degree atrioventricular block and ST-segment elevation.

SECOND-DEGREE ATRIOVENTRICULAR BLOCKS

The term *second-degree AV block* is used when one or more, but not all, sinus impulses are blocked from reaching the ventricles. Because the SA node generates impulses normally, each P wave will occur at a regular interval across the rhythm strip (i.e., all P waves will plot through on time), although a QRS complex won't follow every P wave. This finding suggests that the atria are being depolarized normally, but not every impulse is being conducted to the ventricles (i.e., intermittent conduction). As a result, more P waves than QRS complexes are seen on the ECG.

Second-degree AV block is classified as type I or type II, depending on the behavior of the PR intervals associated with the dysrhythmia.

Second-Degree Atrioventricular Block Type I

Second-degree AV block type I is also known as type I block, Mobitz I, or Wenckebach. With type I AV block, atrial impulses arrive earlier and earlier during the relative refractory period of the AV node, resulting in longer and longer conduction delays and PR intervals, until an impulse arrives during the absolute refractory period and fails to conduct (Issa et al., 2019). The nonconducted impulse appears on the ECG as a P wave with no QRS complex after it. The ECG characteristics of second-degree AV block type I can be summarized as follows (Fig. 7.2):

Rhythm:	Ventricular irregular; atrial regular (i.e., P waves plot through on time); grouped beating may be present
Rate:	Atrial rate is greater than the ventricular rate
P waves:	Normal in size and shape; some P waves are not followed by a QRS complex (i.e., more P waves than QRS complexes)
PR interval:	Lengthens with each cycle (although lengthening may be very slight) until a P wave appears without a QRS complex; the PR interval after a nonconducted P wave is shorter than the interval preceding the nonconducted beat
QRS duration:	Usually 0.11 second or less; complexes are periodically dropped

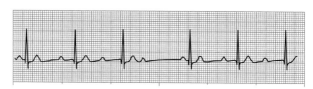

Fig. 7.2 Second-degree atrioventricular block type I at 60 beats/min.

The patient with type I AV block is usually asymptomatic because the ventricular rate often remains nearly normal, and cardiac output is not significantly affected. If the heart rate is slow and serious signs and symptoms occur because of the slow rate, apply a pulse oximeter, administer oxygen (if indicated), obtain the patient's vital signs, and establish intravenous (IV) access. Obtain a 12-lead ECG if doing so will not delay patient treatment. Atropine, administered intravenously, is the drug of choice. Reassess the patient's response and continue monitoring.

Second-Degree Atrioventricular Block Type II

Second-degree AV block type II is also called type II block or Mobitz II AV block. The site of block in second-degree AV block type II is almost always below the AV node. Although second-degree AV block type II is less common than type I, type II is more serious and is a cause for concern because it can progress to a third-degree AV block. The ECG characteristics of second-degree AV block type II include the following (Fig. 7.3):

Rhythm:	Ventricular irregular; atrial regular (i.e., P waves plot through on time)
Rate:	Atrial rate is greater than the ventricular rate; ventricular rate is often slow
P waves:	Normal in size and shape; some P waves are not followed by a QRS complex (i.e., more P waves than QRS complexes)
PR interval:	Within normal limits or prolonged but constant for the conducted beats; the PR intervals before and after a blocked P wave are constant
QRS duration:	Within normal limits if the block occurs above or within the bundle of His; greater than 0.11 second if the block occurs below the bundle of His; complexes are periodically absent after P waves

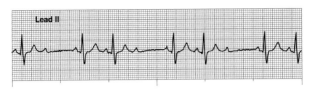

Fig. 7.3 Second-degree atrioventricular block type II at 70 beats/min. (From Aehlert B. *ECG study cards*, St. Louis, 2004, Mosby.)

Because second-degree AV block type II may abruptly progress to third-degree AV block, the patient should be closely monitored for increasing AV block. If the heart rate is slow, and serious signs and symptoms occur because of the slow rate, treatment should include applying a pulse oximeter, administering oxygen (if indicated), obtaining the patient's vital signs, and establishing IV access. Obtain a 12-lead ECG and a cardiology consult. Temporary or permanent pacing may be necessary.

2:1 Atrioventricular Block

With second-degree AV block in the form of 2:1 AV block, there is one conducted P wave followed by a blocked P wave; thus, two P waves occur for every one QRS complex (i.e., 2:1 conduction) (Fig. 7.4). Because there are no two PQRST cycles in a row to compare PR intervals, the 2:1 AV block cannot be conclusively classified as type I or type II. To determine the type of block with certainty, it is necessary to continue close ECG monitoring of the patient until the conduction ratio of P waves to QRS complexes changes to 3:2, 4:3, and so on, which would enable PR interval comparison. The ECG characteristics of 2:1 AV block can be summarized as follows:

Rhythm:	Ventricular regular; atrial regular (P waves plot through on time)
Rate:	Atrial rate is twice the ventricular rate
P waves:	Normal in size and shape; every other P wave is not followed by a QRS complex (i.e., more P waves than QRS complexes)
PR interval:	Constant
QRS duration:	May be narrow or wide; complexes are absent after every other P wave

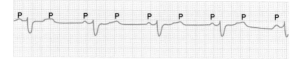

Fig. 7.4 2:1 atrioventricular block. (From Pappano AJ, Wier WG. *Cardiovascular physiology*, ed 11, Philadelphia, 2019, Elsevier.)

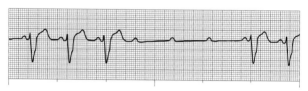

Fig. 7.5 An example of advanced second-degree atrioventricular block. (From Aehlert B. *ECG study cards*, St. Louis, 2004, Mosby.)

If the QRS complex measures 0.11 second or less, the block is likely to be located within the AV node and a form of second-degree AV block type I. A 2:1 AV block associated with a wide QRS complex (i.e., more than 0.11 second) is usually associated with a block below the AV node; thus, it is usually a type II block. The emergency management procedures for 2:1 AV block are those of type I or type II block previously described.

Advanced Second-Degree Atrioventricular Block

The terms advanced or high-grade second-degree AV block may be used to describe three or more consecutive P waves at a normal rate that are not conducted. For example, with 3:1 AV block, every third P wave is conducted (i.e., followed by a QRS complex); with 4:1 AV block, every fourth P wave is conducted (Fig. 7.5).

Because of the frequency with which impulses from the SA node to the Purkinje fibers are blocked, the presence of advanced AV block is a cause for concern, and the development of third-degree AV block should be anticipated.

THIRD-DEGREE ATRIOVENTRICULAR BLOCK

With third-degree AV block, the site of block may occur at the level of the AV node, the bundle of His, or distal to the bundle of His. A secondary pacemaker (either junctional or ventricular) stimulates the ventricles; therefore, the QRS may be narrow or wide, depending on the location of the escape pacemaker and the condition of the intraventricular conduction system. ECG characteristics of third-degree AV block include the following (Fig. 7.6):

Rhythm:	Ventricular regular; atrial regular (P waves plot through); no relationship between the atrial and ventricular rhythms (i.e., AV dissociation is present)
Rate:	Ventricular rate is determined by the origin of the escape pacemaker; atrial rate is greater than (and independent of) the ventricular rate
P waves:	Normal in size and shape; some P waves are not followed by a QRS complex (i.e., more P waves than QRS complexes)
PR interval:	None; the atria and the ventricles beat independently of each other, so there is no true PR interval
QRS duration:	Narrow or wide, depending on the location of the escape pacemaker and the condition of the intraventricular conduction system

The patient's signs and symptoms will depend on the origin of the escape pacemaker (i.e., junctional versus ventricular) and the patient's response to a slower ventricular rate. If the patient is symptomatic as a result of the slow rate, treatment should include applying a pulse oximeter and administering oxygen (if indicated), obtaining the patient's vital

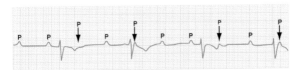

Fig. 7.6 Third-degree atrioventricular block; P waves are marked to show the dissociation between P waves and the QRS complexes. (From Pappano AJ, Wier WG. *Cardiovascular physiology*, ed 11, Philadelphia, 2019, Elsevier.)

signs, establishing IV access, and obtaining a 12-lead ECG. IV administration of atropine may be tried. If the disruption in AV nodal conduction is caused by increased parasympathetic tone, the administration of atropine may be effective in reversing excess vagal tone and improving AV node conduction. Other interventions that may be used in the treatment of third-degree AV block include epinephrine or dopamine IV infusions, or transcutaneous pacing. Frequent patient reassessment is essential. Most patients with third-degree AV block have an indication for permanent pacemaker placement.

REFERENCES

Issa, Z. F., Miller, J. M., & Zipes, D. P. (2019). Atrioventricular conduction abnormalities. In Z. F. Issa, J. M. Miller, & D. P. Zipes (Eds.), *Clinical arrhythmology and electrophysiology: A companion to Braunwald's heart disease* (3 ed., pp. 255–285). Philadelphia, PA: Elsevier.

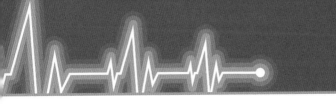

Pacemaker Rhythms 8

PACEMAKER SYSTEMS

A cardiac pacemaker is a battery-powered device that delivers an electrical current to the heart to stimulate depolarization. A pacemaker system consists of a pulse generator and pacing leads. A pacing lead is an insulated wire used to carry an electrical impulse from the pulse generator to the patient's heart. It also carries information about the heart's electrical activity back to the pacemaker. The pulse generator is the power source that houses a battery and electronic circuitry. The circuitry works like a computer, converting energy from the battery into electrical pulses. The pacemaker responds to the information received either by sending a pacing impulse to the heart (i.e., triggering) or by not sending a pacing impulse to the heart (i.e., inhibition).

An artificial pacemaker can be external (a temporary intervention) or implanted.

Permanent Pacemakers and Implantable Cardioverter-Defibrillators

Patients who have chronic dysrhythmias that are unresponsive to medication therapy and that result in decreased cardiac output may require the surgical implantation of a permanent pacemaker or an implantable cardioverter-defibrillator (ICD). Pacemakers and ICDs are called cardiovascular implantable electronic devices (CIEDs).

A permanent pacemaker is used to treat disorders of the sinoatrial (SA) node (e.g., bradycardias), disorders of the AV conduction pathways (e.g., second-degree AV block type II, third-degree AV block), or both, that produce signs and symptoms as a result of inadequate cardiac output.

An ICD can deliver a range of therapies (also called tiered therapy), including defibrillation, antitachycardia pacing (i.e., overdrive pacing), synchronized cardioversion, and bradycardia pacing, depending on the dysrhythmia detected and how the device is programmed. A physician determines the appropriate ICD therapies for each patient.

Pacemaker Leads

Pacemaker lead systems may consist of single, double, or multiple leads. A separate lead is used for each heart chamber paced. The exposed portion of the pacing lead—the electrode—is placed in direct contact with the heart.

A unipolar electrode has one pacing electrode that is located at its distal tip. The negative electrode is in contact with the cardiac tissue, and the pulse generator (located outside the heart) functions as the positive electrode. The pacemaker spike produced by a unipolar lead system is often large because of the distance between the positive and negative electrodes.

A bipolar lead system contains a positive and negative electrode at the distal tip of the pacing lead wire. Most temporary transvenous pacemakers use a bipolar lead system. However, a permanent pacemaker may have either a bipolar or a unipolar lead system. The pacemaker spike produced by a bipolar lead system is smaller than that of a unipolar system because of the shorter distance between the positive and negative electrodes (Fig. 8.1).

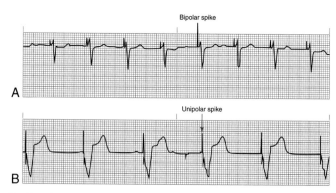

Fig. 8.1 Bipolar and unipolar pacing. **A,** Pacemaker spike produced by a bipolar lead system. **B,** Pacemaker spike produced by a unipolar lead system. (From Urden LD, Stacy KM, Lough ME. *Critical care nursing: diagnosis and management*, ed 9, St. Louis, 2022, Elsevier.)

PACING PRINCIPLES

Pacing, also called pacemaker firing, occurs when the pacemaker's pulse generator delivers energy (milliamperes [mA]) through the pacing electrode to the myocardium. As mentioned earlier, a pacemaker responds to the information received either by sending a pacing stimulus to the heart (i.e., triggering) or by not sending a pacing stimulus to the heart (i.e., inhibiting).

A fixed-rate (asynchronous) pacemaker continuously discharges at a preset rate (usually 70 to 80 impulses/min) regardless of the patient's heart rate or metabolic demands. A demand (synchronous) pacemaker discharges when the patient's heart rate drops below the pacemaker's lower rate limit (also called the base rate), which is expressed in paced pulses per minute (ppm).

Evidence of pacing can be seen as a vertical line or spike on the ECG. Capture is the successful conduction of an artificial pacemaker's impulse through the myocardium, resulting in depolarization. Capture is obtained after the pacemaker electrode is correctly positioned in the heart; with one-to-one capture, each pacing stimulus depolarizes the appropriate chamber. On the ECG, evidence of *electrical capture* can be seen as a pacemaker spike followed by an atrial or a ventricular complex, depending on the cardiac chamber that is being paced. *Mechanical capture* is assessed by palpating the patient's pulse or observing right atrial pressure, left atrial pressure, or pulmonary artery or arterial pressure waveforms.

Single-Chamber Pacemakers

A pacemaker that paces a single heart chamber, either the atrium or ventricle, has one lead placed in the heart. Atrial pacing, achieved by placing the pacing electrode in the right atrium, may be used when the SA node is diseased or damaged, but conduction through the AV junction and ventricles is normal. When spontaneous atrial depolarization does not occur within a preset interval, the pacemaker fires and stimulates atrial depolarization at a preset rate. Atrial stimulation produces a pacemaker spike on the ECG followed by a P wave (Fig. 8.2).

With ventricular demand pacing, the pacemaker electrode is placed in the right ventricle, the ventricle is sensed, and the pacemaker is inhibited when spontaneous ventricular depolarization occurs within a preset interval. The pacemaker will fire and stimulate ventricular

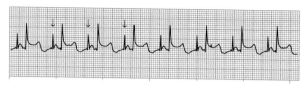

Fig. 8.2 Electrocardiogram of a single-chamber pacemaker with atrial pacing spikes (*arrows*).

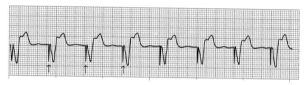

Fig. 8.3 Electrocardiogram of a single-chamber pacemaker with ventricular pacing spikes (*arrows*).

depolarization at a preset rate if spontaneous ventricular depolarization does not occur within this preset interval. Stimulation of the ventricles produces a pacemaker spike on the ECG followed by a wide QRS, resembling a ventricular ectopic beat (Fig. 8.3). The QRS complex is wide because a paced impulse does not follow the heart's normal conduction pathway.

Dual-Chamber Pacemakers

A dual-chamber pacemaker is the most common type of implanted pacemaker. It uses two leads: one lead is placed in the right atrium and the other in the right ventricle.

An optimal sequential pacemaker, also called a physiologic or universal pacemaker, is a type of dual-chamber pacemaker used when the SA node is intact but AV conduction is impaired. The pacemaker is programmed to wait between atrial and ventricular stimulation, simulating the usual delay in conduction through the AV node (i.e., the PR interval). The artificial or electronic PR interval is referred to as an AV interval (Fig. 8.4). If spontaneous atrial or ventricular depolarization does not occur within a preset interval, the pacemaker fires and stimulates the appropriate chamber at a preset rate.

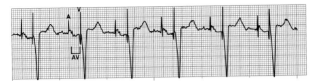

Fig. 8.4 Electrocardiogram of a dual-chamber pacemaker with atrial pacing spikes (*A*), ventricular pacing spikes (*V*). *AV,* Atrioventricular interval.

Biventricular Pacemakers

A biventricular pacemaker has three leads—one lead for each ventricle and one lead for the right atrium. These devices use cardiac resynchronization therapy (CRT) to restore normal simultaneous ventricular contraction, thus improving stroke volume, ejection fraction, cardiac output, and exercise tolerance. CRT, which is indicated for selected patients with moderate to severe heart failure, has been shown to reduce heart failure symptoms and mortality.

PACEMAKER COMPLICATIONS

Problems that can occur with pacing include failure to pace, failure to capture, and failure to sense (e.g., undersensing, oversensing).

Failure to pace, also referred to as failure to fire or failure of pulse generation, is a pacemaker malfunction that occurs when the pacemaker fails to deliver an electrical stimulus at its programmed time. Failure to pace is recognized on the ECG as an absence of pacemaker spikes, even though the patient's intrinsic rate is less than that of the pacemaker, and a return of the underlying rhythm for which pacing was initiated.

Failure to capture is the inability of the artificial pacemaker stimulus to depolarize the myocardium. It is recognized on the ECG by visible pacemaker spikes not followed by P waves (if the electrode is in the atrium) or QRS complexes (if the electrode is in the right ventricle).

Undersensing occurs when the artificial pacemaker fails to recognize spontaneous myocardial depolarization. It is recognized on the ECG by pacemaker spikes that occur within P waves, pacemaker spikes that follow too closely behind the patient's QRS complexes, or pacemaker spikes that appear within T waves.

Oversensing is a pacemaker malfunction that results from inappropriate sensing of extraneous electrical signals. Oversensing is recognized on the ECG as pacemaker spikes at a rate slower than the pacemaker's preset rate or no paced beats even though the pacemaker's preset rate is greater than the patient's intrinsic rate.

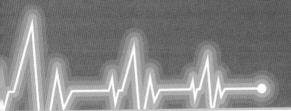

Introduction to the 12-Lead ECG

9

INTRODUCTION

A standard 12-lead electrocardiogram (ECG) provides views of the heart in both the frontal and horizontal planes and views the surfaces of the left ventricle from 12 different angles. Multiple views of the heart can provide useful information including the following:

- Identification of ST-segment and T-wave changes associated with myocardial ischemia, injury, and infarction
- Identification of ECG changes associated with certain medications and electrolyte imbalances
- Recognition of bundle branch blocks (BBBs)

Indications for using a 12-lead ECG include the following:

- Abdominal or epigastric pain
- Assisting in dysrhythmia interpretation
- Chest pain or discomfort
- Diabetic ketoacidosis
- Dizziness
- Dyspnea
- Electrical injuries
- Known or suspected electrolyte imbalances
- Known or suspected medication overdoses
- Right or left ventricular failure
- Status before and after electrical therapy (e.g., defibrillation, cardioversion, pacing)
- Stroke
- Syncope or near syncope
- Unstable patient, unknown etiology

VECTORS

Leads have a negative (−) and positive (+) electrode pole that senses the magnitude and direction of the electrical force caused by the spread of waves of depolarization and repolarization throughout the myocardium.

A *vector* (arrow) is a symbol representing this force. A vector points in the direction of depolarization. Leads that face the tip or point of a vector record a positive deflection on ECG paper. A mean vector identifies the average of depolarization waves in one portion of the heart. The mean QRS vector represents the average magnitude and direction of both right and left ventricular depolarization. The average direction of a mean vector is called the *mean axis*. It is identified only in the frontal plane.

AXIS

An imaginary line joining the positive and negative electrodes of a lead is called the *axis* of the lead. Electrical axis refers to the net direction, or angle in degrees, in which the main vector of depolarization is pointed.

In adults, the normal QRS axis is considered to be between −30 and +90 degrees in the frontal plane. Current flow to the right of normal is called *right axis deviation* (between +90 and ±180 degrees). Current flow in the direction opposite of normal is called *indeterminate*, "no man's land," *northwest* or *extreme right axis deviation* (−90 and ±180 degrees). Current flow to the left of normal is called *left axis deviation* (between −30 and −90 degrees).

Shortcuts exist to determine axis deviation. Leads I and aVF divide the heart into four quadrants. These two leads can be used to quickly estimate electrical axis. In leads I and aVF, the QRS complex is normally positive. If the QRS complex in either or both of these leads is negative, axis deviation is present.

- Normal axis—positive QRS complex in leads I and aVF
- Right axis deviation—QRS negative in lead I and positive in aVF
- Left axis deviation—QRS positive in lead I and negative in aVF
- Northwest—negative QRS complex in leads I and aVF

ACUTE CORONARY SYNDROMES

Acute coronary syndromes (ACSs) are conditions caused by an abrupt reduction in coronary artery blood flow. Partial or intermittent blockage of a coronary artery may result in no clinical signs and symptoms (silent ischemia), unstable angina (UA), non-ST-elevation myocardial infarction (NSTEMI) or, possibly, sudden death. Complete blockage of a coronary artery may result in ST-elevation MI (STEMI) or sudden death. Unstable angina (UA) and NSTEMI are often grouped together as *non-ST-elevation acute coronary syndromes* (NSTE-ACS) because ECG changes associated with these conditions usually include ST-segment depression and T-wave inversion in the leads that face the affected area. Cardiac biomarkers (e.g., troponins) are elevated when an infarction is present. Biomarkers are not elevated in patients with UA because there is no tissue death.

Time is muscle when caring for any patient with an ACS. The region of the heart supplied by the blocked artery is called the *area at risk*. The longer the area at risk is deprived of oxygen and nutrients, the greater the likelihood of permanent damage. Therefore, if myocardium is to be saved, the blockage must be removed before irreversible tissue death occurs. If blood flow is quickly restored, the area at risk can potentially be salvaged. The primary choices for reperfusion therapy are fibrinolysis and percutaneous coronary intervention (PCI).

The area supplied by a blocked coronary artery goes through a sequence of events that have been identified as zones of ischemia, injury, and infarction. Each zone is associated with characteristic ECG changes that affect the shape of the QRS complex, the ST segment, and the T wave (Fig. 9.1). ECG changes of myocardial ischemia, injury, or infarction are considered significant if they are viewed in two or more anatomically contiguous leads. If these ECG findings are seen in leads that look directly at the affected area, they are called *indicative changes*. If findings are seen in leads opposite the affected area, they are called *reciprocal changes*.

INTRAVENTRICULAR CONDUCTION DELAYS

A bundle branch block (BBB) is a disruption in impulse conduction from the bundle of His through either the right or left bundle branch to the Purkinje fibers. A BBB may be intermittent or permanent, complete or incomplete. ECG criteria for BBB recognition include the following:

- QRS duration of 0.12 second or more in adults (if a *complete* right bundle branch block [RBBB] or left bundle branch block [LBBB]); if a BBB pattern is discernible and the QRS duration is between 0.11 and 0.119 second in adults, it is called an *incomplete* right or left BBB.

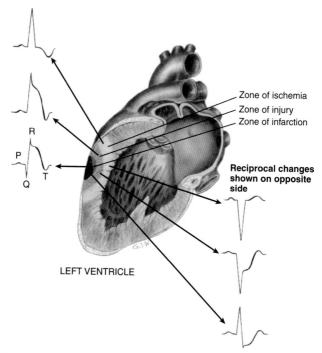

Zone of ischemia
Zone of injury
Zone of infarction

Reciprocal changes shown on opposite side

LEFT VENTRICLE

Fig. 9.1 Zones of ischemia, injury, and infarction showing indicative electrocardiogram changes and reciprocal changes corresponding to each zone. (Modified from Urden LD, Stacy KM, Lough ME. Critical care nursing, ed 7, St. Louis, 2014, Mosby).

(If the QRS is wide but there is no BBB pattern, the term *wide QRS* or *intraventricular conduction delay* is used to describe the QRS.)
- Visible QRS complexes produced by supraventricular activity (i.e., the QRS complex is not a paced beat, and it does not originate in the ventricles).

If a delay or block occurs in one of the bundle branches, the ventricles will not be depolarized at the same time. The impulse first travels down the unblocked branch and stimulates that ventricle. Because of the block, the impulse must then travel from cell to cell through the myocardium (rather than through the normal conduction pathway) to stimulate the other ventricle. The ventricle with the blocked bundle branch is the last to be depolarized.

With BBB, the last ventricle to be depolarized is the ventricle with the blocked bundle branch. Therefore, if it is possible to determine the ventricle that was depolarized last, it becomes possible to determine the bundle branch that was blocked. The final portion of the QRS complex is referred to as the *terminal force*. Examination of the terminal force of the QRS complex reveals the ventricle that was depolarized last and, therefore, the bundle that was blocked. To identify the terminal force, first locate the J point. From the J point, move backward into the QRS and determine whether the last electrical activity produced an upward or downward deflection. An example of the terminal force in both RBBB and LBBB is illustrated in Fig. 9.2. If the right bundle branch is blocked, then the right ventricle will be depolarized last, and the current will be moving from the left ventricle to the right. This will create a positive deflection of the terminal force of the QRS complex in V_1. If the left bundle branch is blocked, the left ventricle will be depolarized last, and the current will flow from right to left. This will produce a negative deflection of the terminal force of the QRS complex seen in V_1. Therefore, to differentiate RBBB from LBBB, look at V_1 and determine whether the terminal force of the QRS complex is a positive or negative deflection. If it is directed upward, an RBBB is present (i.e., the current is moving toward the

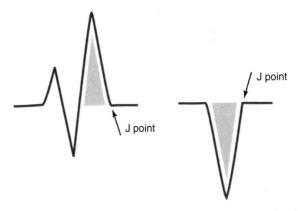

Fig. 9.2 Determining the direction of the terminal force. In lead V_1, move from the J point into the QRS complex and determine whether the terminal portion (last 0.04 second) of the QRS complex is a positive (upright) or negative (downward) deflection. (From Phalen T, Aehlert BJ. *The 12-lead ECG in acute coronary syndromes*, ed 4, St. Louis, 2019, Mosby.)

right ventricle and toward V_1). Conversely, an LBBB is present when the terminal force of the QRS complex is directed downward (i.e., the current is moving away from V_1 and toward the left ventricle).

CHAMBER ABNORMALITIES

Cardiomyopathy is a general term used to describe different heart diseases involving the heart muscle, resulting in abnormal enlargement. *Cardiac enlargement* refers to either dilation of a heart chamber or hypertrophy of the heart muscle (Goldberger et al., 2018). With dilation, stretching of a chamber of the heart muscle occurs, resulting in enlargement of that chamber. Dilation may be acute or chronic. *Cardiac hypertrophy* refers to thickening of the heart muscle, with resultant enlargement of a heart chamber. Hypertrophy is commonly accompanied by dilation. When evaluating the ECG for indications of chamber enlargement, it is essential to check the calibration marker to ensure that it is 10 mm (1 mV) tall.

Atrial Abnormalities

Right atrial abnormality (RAA) produces changes in the initial part of the P wave. The P wave is tall (more than 2.5 mm in height), peaked, and usually of normal duration (Hancock et al., 2009) (Fig. 9.3). The abnormal P waves characteristic of RAA are usually best seen in leads II, III, aVF, and sometimes V_1 (Goldberger et al., 2018).

With left atrial abnormality, the middle and end of the P wave are prolonged because depolarization of the left atrium begins and ends later than right atrial depolarization (Surawicz & Knilans, 2008). Notched P waves are usually visible and correspond with the delay in left atrial activation because the right and left atrial peaks that are usually nearly simultaneous and fused into a single peak become more widely separated (Hancock et al., 2009). Notched P waves are generally most easily seen in the limb leads.

Ventricular Abnormalities

Characteristic ECG changes associated with right ventricular hypertrophy (RVH) include tall R waves in leads V_1 through V_3 and deeper than normal S waves in leads I, aVL, V_5, and V_6 (Sharma & Morrison, 2022). Right axis deviation is usually present, and evidence of RAA may be seen. Left ventricular hypertrophy (LVH) is recognized on the ECG by increased QRS amplitude and changes in the ST segment and T wave. Typically, R waves in leads I, aVL, V_5, and V_6 are taller than normal, and S waves in leads V_1 through V_2 are deeper than normal (Mirvis & Goldberger, 2019). The QRS duration is often increased.

ELECTROLYTE DISTURBANCES

Because electrolyte imbalances may increase cardiac irritability and cause cardiac dysrhythmias, a patient's ECG can be evaluated for evidence of electrolyte disturbances. ECG changes associated with electrolyte imbalances can vary widely from patient to patient.

Potassium

ECG signs of hyperkalemia can include the following:
- Tall, peaked (tented), narrow, symmetric T waves
- P waves decrease in amplitude as potassium level increases
- PR interval and QRS duration increase as potassium level increases

ECG signs of hypokalemia can include the following:
- ST-segment depression
- Decrease in T-wave amplitude
- Prominent U waves; the amplitude of U waves may exceed that of T waves in the same lead with marked hypokalemia
- P-wave amplitude and duration are usually increased
- Slight prolongation of the PR interval
- Increased QRS duration with severe hypokalemia

Calcium

ECG signs of hypercalcemia can include the following:
- Shortening of the ST segment
- Decreased QT-interval duration

ECG signs of hypocalcemia can include the following:
- Lengthening of the ST segment
- Increased QT-interval duration

ANALYZING THE 12-LEAD ELECTROCARDIOGRAM

It is essential to use a systematic method when analyzing a 12-lead ECG. Before beginning an in-depth review, take a moment to "take in" the entire 12-lead and get an overall impression of the tracing. After initially surveying the tracing, consider using the following approach when reviewing a 12-lead ECG:

1. Identify the rate and underlying rhythm. Identify any premature beats and pauses, if present.
2. Estimate the QRS axis using leads I and aVF.
3. Analyze waveforms, segments, and intervals. Before examining waveforms, quickly look at the calibration marker and determine if it is standard, half-standard, or twice the standard. Next, examine each lead, selecting one good representative waveform or complex in each lead. Inspect each waveform, noting any changes in orientation, shape, size, and duration.
4. Examine for evidence of ischemia, injury, and infarction. **I** See **A**ll **L**eads is a commonly used mnemonic to recall the lead groupings when localizing an infarction and predicting which coronary artery is occluded. **I** (inferior) = II, III, aVF; **S** (septal) = V_1, V_2; **A** (anterior) = V_3, V_4; **L** (lateral) = I, aVL, V_5, V_6. Look for the presence of ST-segment displacement (i.e., ST-segment elevation or ST-segment depression).
5. Look for evidence of other conditions. Is there evidence of chamber enlargement, electrolyte imbalances, or conditions that mimic MI (e.g., LVH, left BBB, ventricular rhythm, ventricular paced rhythm)?
6. Interpret your findings.

REFERENCES

Goldberger, A. L., Goldberger, Z. D., & Shvilkin, A. (2018). Atrial and ventricular enlargement. In *Goldberger's clinical electrocardiography: A simplified approach* (9 ed., pp. 50–60). Philadelphia, PA: Elsevier.

Hancock, E. W., Drew, B. J., Mirvis, D. M., Okin, P., Kligfield, P., & Gettes, L. S. (2009). AHA/ACCF/HRS recommendations for the standardization and interpretation of the electrocardiogram: Part V: Electrocardiogram changes associated with cardiac chamber hypertrophy. *J Am Coll Cardiol, 53*(11), 992–1002.

Mirvis, D. M., & Goldberger, A. L. (2019). Electrocardiography. In D. P. Zipes, P. Libby, R. O. Bonow, D. L. Mann, G. F. Tomaselli, & E. Braunwald (Eds.), *Braunwald's heart disease: A textbook of cardiovascular medicine* (11 ed., pp. 117–153). Philadelphia, PA: Elsevier.

Sharma, E., & Morrison, A. R. (2022). Diagnostic tests and procedures in the patient with cardiovascular disease. In E. J. Wing & F. J. Schiffman (Eds.), *Cecil essentials of medicine* (10 ed., pp. 24–42). Philadelphia, PA: Elsevier.

Surawicz, B., & Knilans, T. K. (2008). Atrial abnormalities. In *Chou's electrocardiography in clinical practice* (6 ed., pp. 29–44). Philadelphia, PA: Saunders.

Index

Note: Page numbers followed by *f* indicate figures, *t* indicate tables and *b* indicate boxes.